the *palace* within you

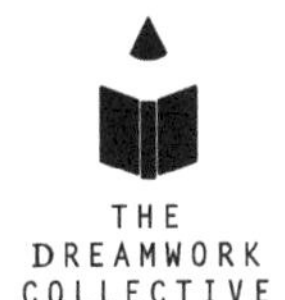

THE
DREAMWORK
COLLECTIVE

This edition was published by The Dreamwork Collective
The Dreamwork Collective LLC, Dubai, United Arab Emirates
thedreamworkcollective.com

Printed and bound in the United Arab Emirates
Cover and design: Kasia Piątek

Text © Nigora Normatova, 2021
ISBN 978-9948-8719-2-7

the *palace* within you

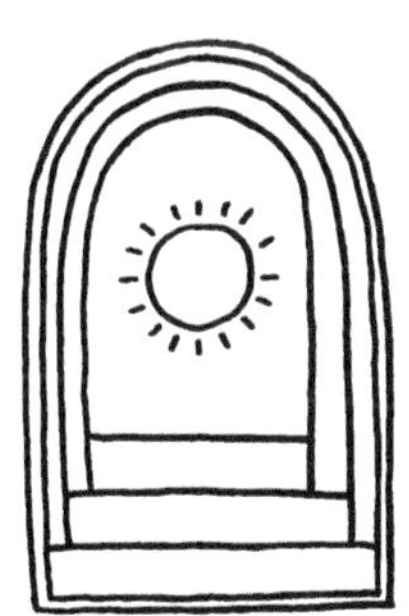

Nigora Normatova

I dedicate this book to my grandmother,
whose smile I will never forget,
whose kindness touched humans and animals,
whose hard work is respected beyond her living days.
I wish I had more time with you.
I miss you so much.

TABLE OF CONTENTS

INTRODUCTION

My parents named me Nigora when I was born in Tajikistan in 1989 because the name means "vision". They had lived in an oppressed era but felt that things were changing and that, with the birth of their third daughter, they would see and experience the world in a different light. And they did.

When I was two, we had to leave Tajikistan due to the civil war. We moved to Moscow, where I was brought up until I was thirteen years old. I have very fond memories of my time in Moscow and always see that place as my home. I was sent to a boarding school in Surrey, England where I spent five years absorbing the British culture at a core level, eventually graduating from the University of Edinburgh in 2011.

After I graduated, I experimented with jobs in different industries ranging from logistics to restaurant management to private equity to IVF to various other start-ups. It was only when I turned twenty-five that I realised I was not living the life I was supposed to. I was not the person I wanted to be or had envisioned when I was little.

I fell into a deep pit of sadness, misery, and pain, and there I stayed until I was advised to carry out a detox and learn to love myself. "Detox?" "Love myself??" These words did not exist in my vocabulary. I had no idea what detox meant, and the idea of loving myself sounded so self-centred and arrogant. Yet I listened, and I tried, and I felt positive results almost immediately.

What did I change? I adopted conscious eating habits, more movement, more free writing, surrounded myself with like-minded people, and started loving and respecting myself more and more. When I noticed the transformation within me, I thought to myself: "I must share this message with the world!" And this is when I started my studies to become a Certified Health Coach, a course that initiated my journey and allowed me to become a stronger, brighter person for all the people I wanted to help and transform.

Later on, I got my hatha yoga, personal trainer, and kundalini yoga qualifications. I also became a Face Fitness trainer in order to empower women with a natural set of skills to induce graceful ageing. And finally, my most recent graduation from Lifestyle Prescriptions University qualifies me as an LP Health Coach looking at brain-organ-mind anatomy to resolve chronic health and emotional issues by tackling the root cause.

I published my first book, *Wake Up! Stop Snoozing on Your Health*, in February 2017, followed by the German version in February 2018. I even travelled to Germany and Austria for the book tour to talk to hundreds of people about health, in German!

Today, through my online platform www.eatthesunglobal.com, I work with many people to improve their lifestyle and health and empower them with knowledge and confidence. Life is a real treat now, and it can only get better. I am so thankful to my strong body for allowing me to do all the things that I do and allowing me to shine bright every day.

Life can be a treat for you, too—when your body is strong, when your mind is grateful, and when your home is your palace within.

My goal in writing this book is to assist and guide you to lead a sustainable healthy lifestyle. The book is divided into three parts.

The first part talks about the importance of thinking about your home environment; in the second part you learn about hidden toxins in the home and what to use instead; and in the third part there is a five-week program where I guide you on how to cleanse and rejuvenate every corner of your soon-to-be palace.

I realised I needed to write this book when I began to understand the impact of our home environment on our health, stress levels, and general well-being. As I was writing the pages, I kept recollecting the home environment I grew up in and the environments my clients lived in before they came to me, and it all started to make sense. I'm so excited for you to work your way through this book to find your palace—your healthy home.

If you've noticed any health concerns, lifestyle imbalances, sleep problems, fatigue, mood swings, or even mild depression, my immediate advice to you would be to start the healing of your home. I don't mean inviting someone to whisper mysterious words into the corners of each room; I mean heal your home by clearing out toxic products and taking nourishing, sustainable, health-conscious steps. That may sound a bit overwhelming, but keep reading, and you may be pleasantly surprised at how simple this can be to do.

Our home is where we rest, repair, reenergize, and rekindle; thus, I strongly believe that a positively charged environment can enhance your health, your mood, and your relationships. Of course, I can't guarantee that health concerns will be eliminated after you complete the five-week program to detox and nourish your home, but what I can guarantee is your increased awareness to make independent conscious steps toward a healthier home.

I always say: "My home is my temple; please leave your slippers outside." In other words, leave all the unnatural and toxic items outside, and keep your home holy, free from intruders that damage your physical and mental state.

From the ingredients in your kitchen to the cleaning products and even the clutter in the rest of your home, everything affects the energy and health of every member of your household. Decreasing the use of plastic, adding plants, decluttering, and protecting yourself from radiation exposure all contribute to increasing the life of your home, and that, in return, will increase the life and energy in you.

As we aim for a healthy, harmonious home, we also focus on sustainability and protecting our environment. With every small action, we contribute to the bigger picture, and even more, we set an example and raise the awareness of people around us.

I recommend that you read the whole book first before making any changes. Trust me, it will all make sense soon. And as you start implementing the changes, you can share your experience on Instagram by using the hashtag #thepalacewithinyou, or tagging my account @nigoranormatova_. I would love to hear from you and cheer you on.

I'm very happy you're here, and I'm even happier that together we will create a ripple effect of harmony out into the world.

Our home is
where we rest,
repair, reenergize,
and rekindle.

Part 1

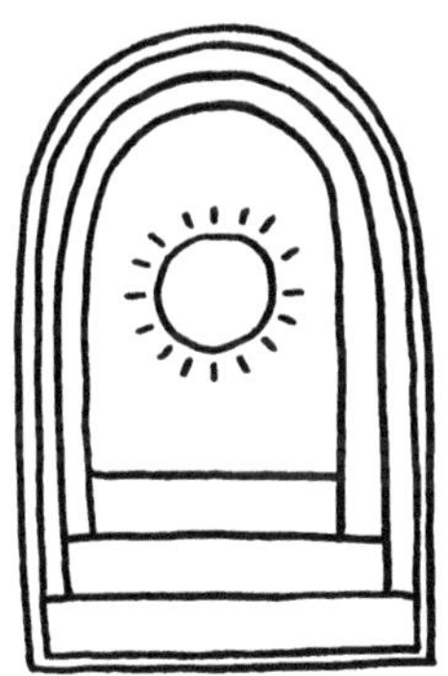

YOU ARE THE KEY

As a health coach, I've worked with many different types of people: young professionals with no family commitments, single mothers, married couples, teenagers, and even kids. Most of them suffer from one or many health issues, whether it's digestive issues or obesity, chronic fatigue or insomnia, high cholesterol, gout, or hypertension. The common element for all is that they haven't connected their dietary choices with their health concern, or their home environment with their general well-being. Unfortunately, many never question the diagnosis they've been slapped with, or the constant feeling of being bloated, or their poor quality of sleep. Instead, they feel cranky and moody because their mother or father experienced the same and so they believe it's inevitable that they will have to start taking medication. And so the chain of "it's normal to be sick and take medication" goes from one generation to another.

When a client starts working with me, we can break that chain. I can teach them how to listen to their body and give them suggestions on how to improve their lifestyle. Soon enough, they realise it is possible to feel healthy and energetic, to have a healthy body shape, and, most importantly, to be pain free. When I realized that I wouldn't be able to individually coach everyone who needed help, I wrote my first book, *Wake Up!*, which then took its own journey to help thousands of individuals.

Why are so many of us so sick? What's the root cause? Is it the effects of a flawed education system? Is it the prescribing of too many pills for any small reason so pharmaceutical companies can make big money? Or is it our fast-pace society, where we need to get things done "yesterday"? Or have we stopped thinking for ourselves and fallen under the influence of crude brainwashing marketing schemes by food industries? And if the answers to some or all of these questions is yes, what then is the key component that needs to be corrected to produce an everlasting healthy effect on generations to come? What is the root cause of our sickness or well-being?

Don't get me wrong; my plan isn't to change the education system, influence the food industry, or even challenge big pharma or big politics. The solution isn't even with them. It is with you. And that's my plan: to empower you with knowledge, tools, and simple strategies so you can take conscious steps toward a healthy home and sustainable lifestyle.

All my clients, no matter their background, had a reckless attitude toward their health and nutrition mainly because of the way they had been brought up. Their parents weren't to blame, nor the parents of their parents, and so on. In fact, there is no time or space or need to identify who is to blame; just realise that you now have the power to give the best love and care to yourself and your loved ones. This love and care start right at home, in your nest, right where you eat, sleep, and rest. In this book, you'll receive guidance on simple ways you can enhance your "nest" and lifestyle from all angles of life, so that you can find that Palace within You.

If you take responsibility for your own well-being, you will gain power, confidence, and the understanding that you can trigger a shift in yourself and set an example to people around you. My kundalini yoga teacher once told me that in order to help others, you first cleanse yourself, ignite the light within you, and allow that light to shine upon others. Be the "lighthouse in the middle of a dark ocean".

Your high energy and strong healthy body will encourage your partner to follow your footsteps. Your mindful way of managing your home and creating a sustainable effect into the future will inspire your friends to emulate you. And your positive and healthy guidance will be remembered and echoed by your children when building their lives and creating their homes. And that's how, hand in hand, you and I will build healthy generations to come.

You are the key to your health, and a healthy home is a very inviting place for positive thoughts, love, and prosperity. You are the key to healthy future generations. You are the trigger that I have been searching for to spark the mind shift in generations to come.

Perhaps all I'm trying to do is ask for your help. Help me spread the message of the importance of a healthy home and a sustainable lifestyle. As you are the key to your healthy household, you are the key to this mission being complete.

Reflections

Before we start learning about how to create a healthy home and which actions to take toward achieving that, it's useful to analyse the home you live in now, and your perception of a healthy environment. Take your time answering these questions. This is simply for you to identify and assess the areas you would want to work on more in your current "nest".

What are the five characteristics of your home now?

What five characteristics would you want to add to your home?

Are there items in your home that are associated with
negative feelings, e.g., sadness, anger, frustration?

How would you describe the products you use to clean
your house?

How would you describe your kitchen and the ingredients
you use?

What about the products you use on your skin?
Are they toxin free? Tested on animals?

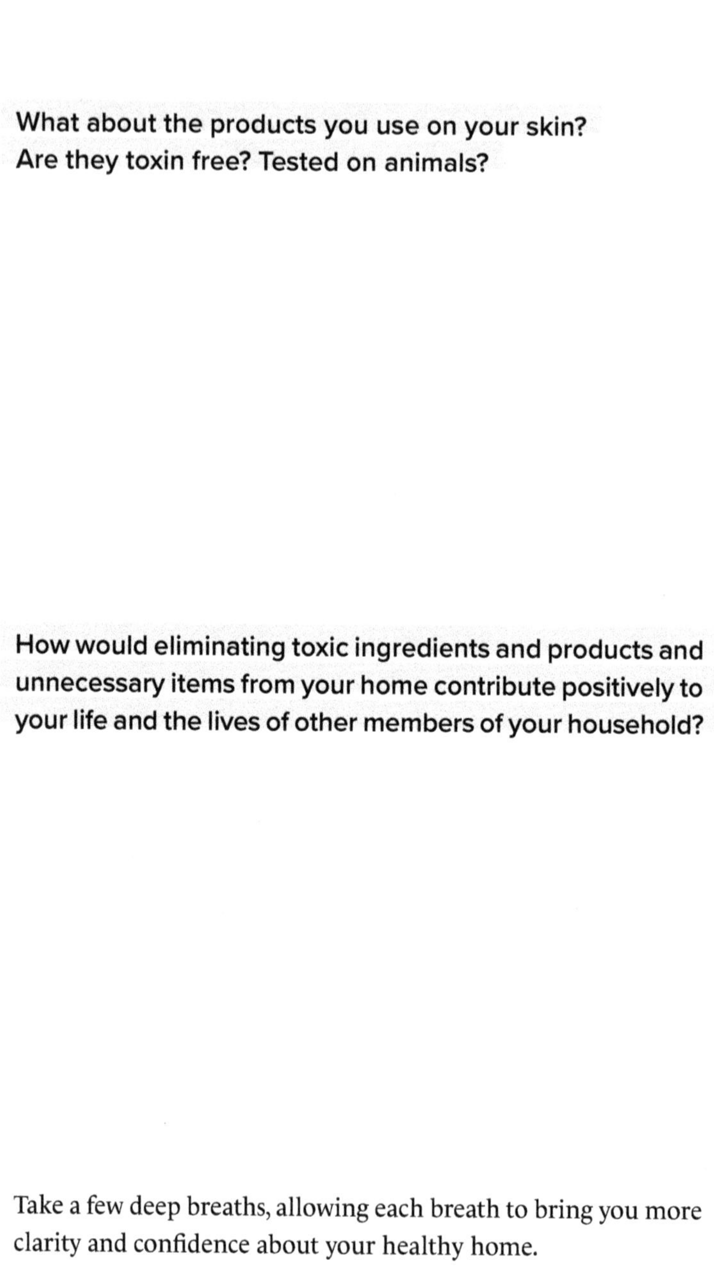

How would eliminating toxic ingredients and products and
unnecessary items from your home contribute positively to
your life and the lives of other members of your household?

Take a few deep breaths, allowing each breath to bring you more
clarity and confidence about your healthy home.

Now, if you didn't have any constraints with money, time, or location, describe your ideal home, highlighting every detail: furniture, plants, food, energy in the home, who you live with, and your daily lifestyle.

YOUR HOME ENVIRONMENT

Some people pay no attention to their house, seeing it only as a place to sleep. This can be especially true of people in big cities who are often the ones always in a rush, never revitalised, always tired, struggling to slow down and to become more mindful. Could there be a connection between such a "go-go-go" lifestyle and the disconnection between themselves and their body? Initial health concerns associated with such a way of living could come in the form of allergies, chronic fatigue, digestive issues, high cholesterol, and even mild depression. After some time, these initial health issues might grow into more serious problems, due to no time to treat the first symptoms. Quality of life becomes even poorer and the list of medications becomes even longer, and the root cause of all the issues was a combination of high stress, inadequate rest, improper nutrition, and lack of mindful activities. Let's break it down one by one.

HIGH STRESS

Stress is the number one cause for any sickness to knock on your door. Stress increases the acidity and inflammation of the body, which is a perfect formula for a health breakdown. You're probably fully aware of the negative side effects of stress, but have you thought about the connection between your stress levels and your home environment? Imagine this scenario: You had a tough day at work, you return home, and your home is a toxic combination of dust, mess, unhealthy food, poor air quality, and overexposure to radiation. How might you feel? Can you see yourself finding peace and relaxation in such an environment? Hardly. Can you see yourself enjoying several hours of deep, restorative sleep? Not at all. Thus, the stress levels in your body stay the same, and you wake up the next day still feeling tired. Sound familiar? And when we feel stressed, anxious, or unhappy in our own environment, any existing issues are heightened, causing even more stress to the body and subsequently leading to health concerns and body discomforts.

INADEQUATE REST

You might be falling asleep, but the question is, how many hours of deep sleep are you getting? When your body is in deep sleep, your body repairs and restores itself. If your stress levels are high, a stress hormone called cortisol will interfere with the secretion of the sleep hormone melatonin, which is responsible for your sleep-wake cycle. Night after night, you get less sleep, get more fatigued during the day, and get stuck in a vicious cycle with caffeine, sugar, and sweets to keep you awake. Furthermore, radiation exposure from your Wi-Fi box, your mobile phone, or even the TV can significantly disturb your sleep.

IMPROPER NUTRITION

When your grocery shopping consists of buying foods from the middle aisles of the supermarket, you're more likely to "junk up" your body regularly. My simple rule of thumb is "If you buy it, you'll eat it. So, don't buy it." Purchasing foods processed, packaged, sweetened, salted, in boxes, cans, and packets will not only heighten existing inflammation and acidity in your body but also deplete it of essential vitamins and minerals. When your cells don't receive the nutrition to function 100 percent, your body reacts, making you feel lethargic, bloated, anxious, lazy, and inactive, which, after some time, can lead to more serious health concerns. Treating your kitchen as a temple, as a holy place where your body regularly receives the nourishment it needs and deserves, would give you the flexibility and the guilt-free opportunities to have occasional "cheat meals" during outings.

LACK OF MINDFUL ACTIVITIES

Who wants to take part in sporting activities or slow down in a meditation routine when their body is going through stress, malnutrition, lethargy, or any type of discomfort? Or perhaps the environment of their home isn't inviting for them to light a candle or roll out a yoga mat. Many adults think they're too old for journaling, and children sometimes feel they are too "cool" for colouring books. Instead, both generations feel drawn to scroll down their phones, watch TV, or stare at iPads. These activities are perceived by many people as relaxation or switching off; however, this type of scrolling and staring activates the brain cells, exposes them to radiation, worsens posture, and some people even get joint pain in their left or right hand due to holding/working with the phone all the time! Introducing mindful activities will slow you down and allow you to live in the present moment. But before you take that step, first create a home environment where activities of this type will flood in without much effort, you nourish your body in your healthy "holy" kitchen, and you enjoy long hours of quality deep sleep.

If you could enhance all these elements through creating a beautiful pure environment in your home, how do you think you would feel? Rested, energetic, positive, and even influential! You'd be contributing to the bigger picture by leading a sustainable lifestyle and acting as an inspiration to your family, children, and friends. You may even experience the beautiful mind shift from "what about me?" to "what about them?"

When I took the steps to enhance my home to become healthy, sustainable, energizing, and a place for rest and repair, I created more space for positive energy to come in, whether it was in the form of new waves of creativity, new meaningful friendships, or even new projects. I'm certain that once you implement the steps from this book, not only your health but many other areas of your life will improve, too.

I'm with you all the way.

Reflections

Take time to analyse your current stress levels, sleep quality and the ways you rest, your nutrition, and what types of activity you're involved in.

Current Stress Level:
High / Medium / Low

NUTRITION

Quantity of processed and packaged foods

Do you consider your kitchen a healthy place?

Do you like to cook?

QUALITY OF SLEEP AND REST

How many hours do you sleep?

Do you wake up during the night?

Do you wake up full of energy?

Do you rest during the day? How?

ACTIVITIES

What types of activity are you already involved in?

What types of activity would you like to be involved in?

What obstacles are preventing you from taking part in activities?

THE PALACE WITHIN YOU

The significance of my home and sustainable lifestyle, for me, is paramount. By taking measures to create a palace outside of me, I naturally create a palace within me. I choose the word "palace" not because I live in a massive castle but because it signifies grandeur, royalty, importance—meanings I want you to bring into your home as well. Whether you live in a small apartment or a big house, the "palace" can only be found when you invest attention and energy into every corner of your home. Most of the time, the environment of your home is a reflection of your internal state. Review the questions you answered in the previous section and try to determine if there's a connection between your stress levels and the state of your bedroom, or your health status and the state of your kitchen.

Instead of digging deep and changing your internal state, let's start by taking a simpler step by enhancing the environment of your house. This will influence your internal state. This is when you find the palace within you.

When I ask my clients about their home environment, they don't quite understand the question or the relevance of it, yet these same people are experiencing health concerns, lack the motivation to exercise or cook, have very low levels of joy, find little satisfaction in their job, and so on. When I carried out a health coaching program where we worked on their home environments, on their cooking skills, on their eating habits and physical activities, suddenly, all the other parts of their life got heightened, too: the job didn't seem so bad and they found themselves feeling more creative and joyful. One of the tools we used was the Circle of Life, completing it before and after the program.

And this is my next invitation for you. Please look at the Circle of Life and mark a dot on each line of each life element to indicate your level of satisfaction. Placing a dot closer to the circle centre shows dissatisfaction, whereas placing a dot toward the periphery shows satisfaction. Connect the dots and see where you're out of balance.

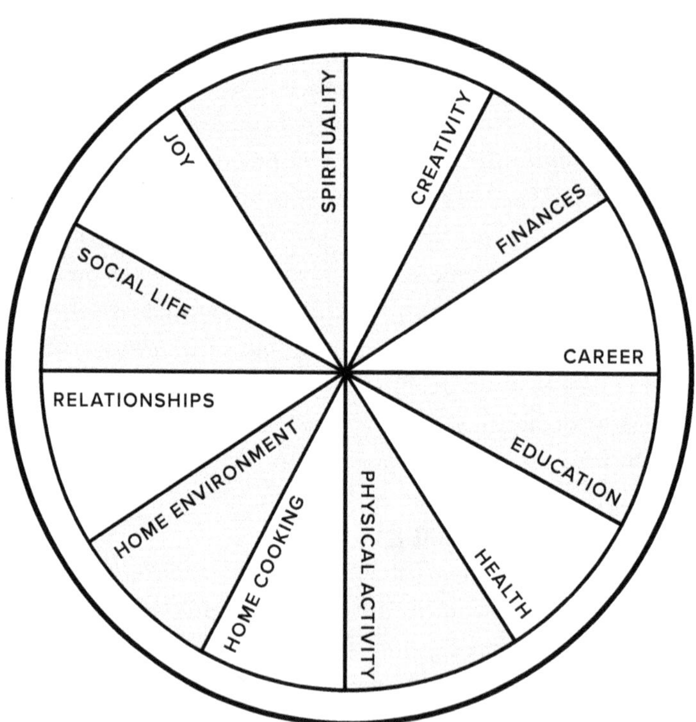

Once you've filled out the circle, ask yourself this question: A car has four wheels, and if one of the wheels happened to be your Circle of Life, how far would the car go? Perhaps the journey would be either very bumpy or there would be no journey at all. And this is when you might realise the imbalances, flaws, and aspects of your life that have been neglected. This is a great exercise to come back to every so often to check in with yourself. I strongly recommend filling out the Circle of Life once again after you complete the five-week program to detox and nourish your home. You can find a blank Circle of Life on page 209. One note: Try not to look at the first one you did before you fill out the second.

Usually, improving one's home environment, home cooking, and physical activity has a ripple effect on all the other elements in the circle.

There's so much within you; not only cells and organs but a palace of strength, courage, love, kindness, self-care, and so much creativity. More often than not, we live out of a "shack", struggling with each day and wondering "why me?" By shack, obviously I don't mean a physical shack but living a lifestyle that holds the energy of a shack: neglected, cluttered, unhealthy, and toxic. We aren't here to suffer; we're here to live, thrive, and experience life in all its colours. We're here to live in a palace that we create for ourselves.

How to do it? Start by detoxing and nourishing your home. Once your home is cleared from all the toxins and nourished with goodness instead, your environment will support you adopting healthy eating habits, exercising, taking part in mindful activities, and becoming a more responsible conscious inhabitant of this planet.

And you'll start living your life from the palace within you.

Let's now explore each part of a home and identify the culprits for our discomforts.

Part 2

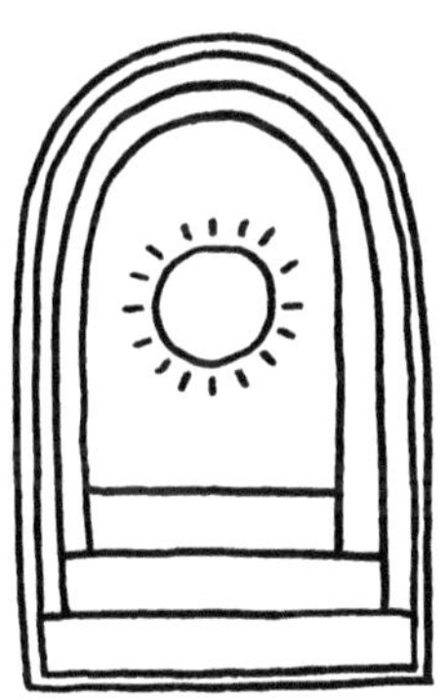

THE KITCHEN

I believe that health starts in the kitchen. When I worked with clients offline, I had the opportunity to visit their kitchens. By opening the fridge and the cupboards, I could immediately figure out why my client was suffering from joint pain, obesity, or fatigue. Cupboards were filled with table salt, white sugar, processed oils, grains, and various packaged "foods". The fridge was filled with bottled salad dressings, fizzy drinks, jams, processed foods, and so on. Sometimes, the kitchen was empty, with only a couple of alcoholic beverages in the fridge, which can be even worse than a kitchen with the wrong foods. Of course, I didn't blame the client. How were they meant to know the health consequences of products that are promoted to them so cleverly? I then helped them carry out a kitchen clearance or kitchen enhancement, educating them about every single product and transforming their kitchen into a health-promoting one rather than a health-degrading one.

I invite you to do the same! Let's go through a typical kitchen and identify the damaging products and ingredients. We can also learn the possible negative effects of them on your health and identify some healthy alternatives. As we go through each ingredient, I want you to take a moment and answer how often you use this product and whether you're ready to throw it away and substitute it with a proposed alternative.

VEGETABLE OILS

"Vegetable" oil is not a very accurate label for sunflower oil, safflower oil, corn oil, and soy oil because these oils aren't actually made from vegetables but extracted from the seeds of vegetables and, sometimes, from what aren't even vegetables. The process of producing the oil involves refining, bleaching, and degumming with high heat and chemical solvents. These oils become processed and chemically reactive before they even reach your kitchen. When used for cooking, they're typically subjected to even more heat and, as a result, contain even more of what are known as free radicals, which attack your body cells and increase the risk of heart disease.[1]

Canola oil? you may ask. Did you know that the real name for this oil is "lower erucic acid rapeseed"? Because this name seemed too offensive to use for marketing purposes, they came up with "can", because it's a Canadian invention, and "ola" for oil. The extraction from the rapeseed plant undergoes the same high-heat process with various chemical solvents, creating a refined oil with traces of trans fats. To top it all off, 90 percent of canola oil comes from genetically modified rapeseed.[2]

You can further investigate vegetable oils by reading the book *Eat Fat Get Thin* by Dr Mark Hyman. But the descriptions here of the oils are quite clear and scary enough, if you ask me! Seemingly so innocent and so commonly used, they can be so health damaging. Which oils are used when we dine out is beyond our control; however, we can certainly avoid using vegetable oils at home.

HEALTHY OIL ALTERNATIVES
olive oil, coconut oil, avocado oil, ghee butter

Every client I work with is surprised to hear the truth about the vegetable oils that they and their families have been using for decades. However, after some reflection, many of them realize their parents also suffered from cardiovascular problems, high cholesterol, or diabetes. They had thought that these health problems ran in their families. But what really "ran in the families" was the vegetable oils that clogged up their arteries and left them diseased.

The most nutritious alternative would be olive oil, to be used for salads and dressings only, not for cooking as it has a low smoke point (the temperature at which the oil oxidises, creating free radicals). Delicious, and nutritious due to its antioxidant composition, olive oil is excellent for heart health,[3] anti-inflammatory, and even antimicrobial. Due to the fragile nature of the polyphenols, the antioxidant found in olive oil, it's best to store olive oil in a dark cool place and consume it within two months.

Coconut oil, which is highly digestible and suitable for cooking, is known for its unique chemical composition that can assist in treating cardiovascular disease,[4] boosting the immune system, and increasing energy levels. Moreover, unlike olive oil, coconut oil escapes rancidity, stays nutritionally potent, and can be used within two years.

Along with coconut and olive oils, the next healthiest oil to use is avocado oil. Studies show that avocado oil helps with the prevention of diabetes development, high cholesterol, high triglyceride levels, and obesity.[5] It can be used for salads but also for cooking due to its high smoke point. It also helps reduce blood pressure, decreases inflammation in joints, and assists the absorption of other nutrients. According to a study published in the *Journal of Nutrition*, the addition of avocado oil to a salad enhances the absorption of vitamin A (alpha-, beta-carotene and lutein found in carrots, broccoli, spinach, kale, zucchini).[6]

Ghee butter has been around for thousands of years. Originating from India, ghee is clarified butter made from cow's milk. The process, which involves simmering the butter for a very long time, removes milk fats and water, making the butter compatible with high smoke points. Creating a more alkaline state in the body, ghee butter has been used in traditional Indian medicinal practices (Ayurveda science) and has been shown to reduce inflammation, assist digestion and weight loss, build strong bones, and even help you absorb fat-soluble vitamins such as A, D, and E.[7] Some people who suffer from gluten sensitivity, leaky gut, IBS, and Crohn's disease aren't able to absorb vitamin A. Incorporating ghee butter into the diet can definitely improve absorption. Lactose and casein free, ghee butter should be a staple ingredient in all health-conscious homes.

TABLE SALT

I'm not quite sure why table salt was ever invented, because there are so many other nutritional alternatives, but, either way, it's important to understand why table salt is a big "no no" and must not be used at home. Table salt is 97 percent processed sodium chloride and 3 percent various chemicals and additives. Because it is completely refined with ferrocyanide and aluminosilicate chemicals (which most of us wouldn't know how to pronounce!), table salt can lead to greater risk of high blood pressure.[8] Furthermore, the nature of table salt means it holds on to liquid, leading to water retention in the body, which consequently leads to problems such as gout, diabetes, and obesity. Also, the addition of iodine to table salt means that people can suffer from overiodization, which can lead to thyroid problems.

We require salt for complete mineral nutrition, but the type of salt we choose matters.[9] It's time to throw away the refined table salt and turn to Mother Nature.

HEALTHY SALT ALTERNATIVES
Flake sea salt, celtic sea salt, himalayan pink salt

As already mentioned, we need salt because of its mineral content. Here, you may think sea salt would be the best alternative to table salt; however, it is not. Over the years, the seas and oceans have become polluted with plastic residues and chemicals from oil spills, and it is no longer advisable to use sea salt. However, Himalayan pink salt can serve the purpose of enriching your body with essential trace minerals, including calcium, potassium, magnesium, and trace amounts of zinc, manganese, and iron. Before you go salting all your food, I recommend carrying out what I call a "salt test": go without Himalayan salt for 10 days, and on day 11, salt your food for lunch and dinner, and check the effect on your body on day 12: you may notice weight fluctuation, water retention, digestive issues, or skin breakouts. If you experience no issues at all, your relationship with Himalayan pink salt has passed the test. Furthermore, be very aware that nearly all packaged foods contain salt—the "naughty" kind of salt.

SUGAR

It's the scariest product ever invented! My teeth literally go numb every time I think about sugar. Did you know that sugar-sweetened diets can be compared to drug addiction, because they both produce a similar effect on the brain?[10] The habits of adding a few spoons of sugar to tea or coffee, sprinkling it over strawberries, or even adding sugar to porridge to encourage kids to eat it are all destructive for the whole body, head to toe. Sugar can negatively impact brain function, cause non-alcoholic fatty liver disease to develop, cause gut issues and metabolic disorders,[11] make the body more prone to diabetes,[12] and accelerate cell aging.[13]

The reason behind hyperactivity in children or their difficulty to focus and concentrate at school may be due to the "sugar rush" that's playing out in their body. Unfortunately, so many food products contain sugar, we unconsciously keep sugar-coating our tongue, meaning anything not sugared starts to taste bland. We lose sensitivity in our taste buds, and as a result, feel the need to enhance our food with even more sugar, a vicious cycle that's very hard to get out of. It usually takes a minimum of seven days without any sugar products for the coating on your tongue to be cleared and your palate to readjust. Seven days is a very long time for a sugar addict! The statistics on children's diseases are shocking. There has been a 1,000 percent increase in the number of cases of children diagnosed with type 2 diabetes, whereas fifteen years ago, there was only 3 percent of such cases.[14] What has happened in the last fifteen years? Today, you can meet five-year-olds with liver cirrhosis from drinking soda drinks, and there's been a 50 percent increase of heart stroke incidents in children aged five to fourteen.[15]

It isn't the fault of the children, and they won't stop craving and eating sugar, unless their caregivers provide them with the education and a healthy foundation, which starts at home. If they grow up in an environment where sugar isn't the "normal" product of use, this will be seeded into their subconscious mind and allow them to make better choices as they grow up.

The first step to spread awareness is to get to know the subject. So, what is sugar and where does it hide? Sugar (sucrose) is a simple carbohydrate, comprising 50 percent fructose and 50 percent glucose. Glucose is mostly found in carbohydrates and is metabolized in every single cell of the body, whereas fructose is metabolized in the liver, which converts most of it into fat. And when we have a high percentage of fat in our body, the whole system starts to slowly shut down, throwing the body out of balance and affecting the functioning of every organ and cell. We need to be aware of fructose and keep its intake to a minimum. Due to its different metabolic pathway, fructose isn't a preferred source of energy for the brain, the muscles, or the body overall. Here is a chart of ingredients to watch out for on product labels; all are converted into high amounts of fructose in the body and, as a result, can lead to numerous health problems.

Anhydrous dextrose	Agave syrup	Brown sugar
Dextrose	HCFS / Corn syrup	White sugar
Lactose	Pancake syrup	Raw cane sugar
Nectars	Malt syrup	Palm sugar
Maltose	Molasses	Date sugar
Corn syrup solids	Brown rice syrup	Coconut sugar

Most of these ingredients can be found in baked goods, cakes, candy, gum, frozen dairy products (ice cream, frozen yoghurt), biscuits, jarred and canned foods, chocolate spreads, cheese spreads, ketchup, various sauces and dressings, cured meats, and many other packaged products, in order to enhance their shelf life and, of course, taste. In addition, they can be found in energy drinks, packaged juices, and soda drinks. In order to avoid putting yourself and your family at risk, it's important to significantly cut back on these "taste-enhanced" foods and keep what you put into your body natural and wholesome. Besides, there's absolutely no nutritional value in any of them, except the date sugar and coconut sugar, which we'll discuss in the healthy alternative section.

The other side of sugar is to question the natural fructose found in fruits. Although fruits are a great source of vitamins, their fructose content can be quite damaging to the body. Thus, keeping the consumption of fruit to controlled quantities would be safer. It's advised to reduce the consumption of fructose to 25 grams per day.[16] Just imagine, a can of soda (350 ml) contains 40 grams of sugar, more than half of which is fructose. With just that one drink you will have almost reached your sugar consumption limit, yet there's a high chance you will eat other processed foods and perhaps fruits throughout your day, which will add up to even more fructose consumption. And somehow we still get quite surprised when we gain weight or develop some sort of health concern.

Dr Richard Johnson, in his book *The Sugar Fix*, gives us a detailed table showing the amount of fructose in fruits as well as other foods. Please take a look at this table (page 199) and figure out whether your fruit intake exceeds the recommended maximum intake of 25 grams. I would also like to add, if you're on a weight loss journey or trying to combat some health concern (especially digestive issues), it's best to keep your fructose intake to 15 grams or less.

HEALTHY SWEET ALTERNATIVES
Monk fruit sweetener, natural herb stevia, dates, coconut sugar, raw honey, maple syrup

Except for natural stevia and monk fruit sweetener, all of the healthy alternatives also contain fructose, and to the body are no different from sugar, as fructose gets converted to glucose and is used for metabolic fuel. However, the amount of fructose is significantly lower than in all other types of sugar. For example, the fructose in maple syrup is 35 percent compared with 85 percent in agave syrup. Coconut sugar and dates can be used for baking, raw honey and Manuka honey can be added to smoothies, and maple syrup can be drizzled over your pancakes on that one cheat day. Aside from the fructose, dates are a source of fibre and potassium,[17] raw honey is a source of phytochemicals, antioxidants, and electrolytes,[18] and Manuka honey has antioxidant and antibacterial properties and is very effective at treating ulcers and improving overall immune system.[19]

Herb stevia and monk fruit sweetener are completely natural sweeteners with no fructose or calories. Stevia comes from the leaf of a flowering plant and monk fruit sweetener comes from the monk fruit itself. A little bit of it goes a long way to sweeten your baked goods, smoothies, or tea. w so you can indulge without feeling too guilty.

REFINED CARBOHYDRATES
white flour, white bread, white pasta, cereals

For baking cakes, muffins, and breads, and making pancakes or pasta, many households use white flour, which is a processed refined carbohydrate that, when consumed, is broken down into sugar (glucose) in the body. And from the previous section about sugar, we now know that overloading on sugar can be very harmful to our health. The white flour, white bread, white pasta, and breakfast cereals that make a regular appearance on your grocery list are processed foods, and, as they enter the body, they're immediately broken down into the simplest forms of sugar. That's why we refer to them as simple carbohydrates. Simple, refined carbohydrates have been completely stripped of nutritional value.

Unaware that there are alternatives, people tend to stick to white bread, breakfast cereals, and quick pasta meals with canned tomato sauce: very convenient, yet nothing to nourish our health.

HEALTHY FLOUR ALTERNATIVES
buckwheat flour, oat flour, rye flour, spelt flour, almond flour, coconut flour, chickpea flour, sprouted flours, brown rice flour, wholewheat flour

What a selection of flours! Moreover, each one comes with a bag of nutrition and health values, such as lowering cholesterol and blood pressure,[20] assisting weight loss, managing sugar levels,[21] and boosting the immune system. Except for rye and spelt flour, all other flours are gluten free; however, even rye or spelt contain gluten that's easily digested and tolerated in comparison to wheat. With fibre, minerals, and vitamins—and even healthy fats in the case of coconut flour[22]—these flours should be the staple flours in each home.

Also, a separate note on sprouted flours and grains, which could be any grains, legumes, beans, or seeds. The key variation to the flour or grain is that it's sprouted, which triples or quadruples the existing nutritional value of the food,[23] making it even healthier and classified as a superfood. Sprouting occurs by simply germinating the seeds in water for a certain amount of time. This method has been carried out for thousands of years for easy digestion and better absorption of nutrients. I prefer to purchase sprouted flours from organic sources and sprout my own grains. (See page 197 to learn how.)

It's now just a matter of identifying which flours are your favourites, adopting these flours to your favourite recipes, and enjoying your baked goodies guilt free. (See the Recipe section, page 191, for my ways of using my favourite flours.)

HEALTHY BREAD ALTERNATIVES
wholewheat bread, rye bread, spelt bread, sourdough bread

People have a very strong attachment to bread. No matter what culture, bread is a big part of any meal. In fact, according to Dr Douillard, 10,000 to 12,000 years ago, wheat was already domesticated and was the main source of food across the African continent. In his book *Eat Wheat*, he states that we only started hunting for meat 500,000 years ago, whereas we have the genetics for eating wheat, barley, and gluten dating back to three to four million years ago. So why are we trying to get off wheat today? Why are so many people unable to digest wheat? It's because our digestive systems have become very sensitive to anything that's slightly harder to digest, such as wheat products. Some people suffer from celiac disease, which means they must not eat gluten, but most of us have damaged our digestive systems through medication intake, lack of water, processed sugar, alcohol, and lots of junk food. I believe that, three to four million years ago, our diet was a lot more natural than it is today. Repair your digestive system, carry out an elimination diet or my five-week program plan from my book *Wake Up!*, and very soon after, you'll be able to indulge in wholewheat breads or sourdough bread without suffering from bloat or weight gain.

Of course, any type of bread is still a carbohydrate and is broken down into sugar; however, the sugar release is much slower due to the large fibre content in wholegrain bread. And remember, we need carbohydrates; they're our primary source of energy. All we're required to do now is to be smart in our choices and fill our cupboards with the right types of product.

Sourdough bread has become my personal favourite type of bread. I have learned how to bake it myself and have even created an online course to teach the skill to you. Sourdough bread carries a whole bunch of fermented bacteria, which are very beneficial for the diversity of your gut flora. To eat bread without guilt is really one of life's greatest delights, and thanks to the process of sourdough breadmaking, we can finally enjoy bread and have no digestive troubles at all.

HEALTHY PASTA ALTERNATIVES
wholewheat pasta, brown rice pasta, quinoa pasta, buckwheat pasta, black rice noodles, soba noodles

There's a common assumption that pasta is a delicious simple carbohydrate without any nutritional value. However, a good quality pasta can be a source of complex carbohydrates, fibre, and even some minerals, depending on what pasta flour you choose. Making your own pasta at home is another level of cooking skill; however, it's a common skill amongst women in Italy. Homemade pasta is not only more delicious but also very nutritious and, unlike the processed pasta bought from a supermarket shelf, it doesn't spike up sugar levels in the body. If you don't have enough time to make your own pasta, you can certainly find brown rice pasta, wholewheat pasta, and other alternatives to processed wheat pasta. It's important to read the ingredient list on the package to make sure that no refined wheat flour was used. For a homemade pasta recipe where you can get the whole family involved, see page 195.

HEALTHY ALTERNATIVES TO CEREALS / MORNING CORN FLAKES
none or homemade granola

I grew up on cereals and milk. Whether it was corn flakes, chocolate balls, or any other "sugar-loaded" bowl with milk, that was how I started my day. Now I know why I always suffered from a heavy bloated feeling, brain fog, general lethargy, and sugar rushes in addition to being lactose intolerant. I have to admit that boxed cereal is a very easy and convenient food for children and adults alike, but it's also a source of sugar, not ideal to start the day, has no nutritional value, and is quite damaging to the digestive system. An early morning sugar spike every day can lead to an array of unwanted health concerns, one of them being weight gain. Once we gain weight, the body falls out of balance and invites a whole bunch of other unpleasant symptoms. This is the effect of sugar. Whether sugar should be banned from your house is up to you, but how about making a homemade granola and enjoying that with homemade nut milk? Sounds pretty inviting to me! (See recipes for homemade granola and nut milk on pages 175 and 196, respectively.)

WHITE RICE

Did you know that white rice originally grows brown and then undergoes refining and polishing, losing all its minerals and fibre in the process? White rice acts as a simple carbohydrate and when consumed breaks down into sugar, increasing insulin production, which, over time, can lead to weight gain, diabetes, and other cardiovascular problems.[24]

You may be surprised and question how this can be when in the Far East and Middle East, a day doesn't go by without a bowl of white rice at each meal. But what you also need to question is the level of obesity and diabetes in those areas, and the level of their physical activity. When I lived in China, I hardly ever saw overweight people, and in my opinion it's because they are constantly moving, exercising, doing tai chi, or simply walking for miles and miles. The occasional large person is most likely a businessperson who drives a car, sits in an office, and doesn't have time for exercise. Sound familiar?

Of course, white rice is delicious, yet the nutritional value is low. And I believe, most of the time, we eat to nourish our cells to repair, grow, and function, whereas at other times, we can eat for pleasure. Another issue that we face today is the level of arsenic in our inorganic rice.[25] How did it get there? Due to contaminated soil or water, arsenic is taken up by the roots of rice crops and ends up being stored in the grains. Rice is much more predisposed to arsenic uptake than any other grain, as it's one of the only major crops that grows in water-flooded conditions. The solution to reducing arsenic in your diet is to buy rice from organic sources and to rinse the rice several times before cooking.

HEALTHY GRAIN ALTERNATIVES
brown rice, black rice, wild rice, quinoa, buckwheat, millet

The common element between these healthy alternative grains is that they're complex carbohydrates that release sugar slowly, triggering a slow release of insulin. Carbohydrates are the first source of energy for our body, essential for us to feel good and stay active. Diets low in carbohydrates can lead to body fat loss, but such diets aren't sustainable. Therefore, I suggest you choose your carbohydrates wisely and fill your cupboards with these smart alternatives. Enjoying carbohydrates without feeling guilty is most likely to be a heavenly treat for people used to dieting, especially after you read their benefits.

Brown rice	Source of manganese, selenium, magnesium, phosphorous, B vitamins, fibre, protein Low glycaemic index Supports heart health, bone development, immune system defence, decreases cholesterol levels
Black rice	Source of antioxidants, protein, iron, fibre, and B vitamins Supports heart health, assists the detoxification of the body, regulates sugar levels, improves digestive health
Wild rice	Source of antioxidants, protein, iron, fibre, and B vitamins Supports heart health, assists the detoxification of the body, regulates sugar levels, improves digestive health
Quinoa	Contains all 8 fatty amino acids making it a complete protein Source of B vitamins, iron, zinc, potassium, calcium, and vitamin E Supports kidney, heart, and lung function
Buckwheat	Source of protein, zinc, copper, manganese, potassium High in soluble fibre, slowing the rate of glucose absorption Aids with control of concerns such as hypertension, obesity, constipation
Millet	Source of protein, fibre, magnesium, antioxidants Aids with control of concerns such as diabetes and inflammation

Source: "The Nutrition Source," Harvard School of Public Health, www.hsph.harvard.edu, 2018

These grains are very easy to cook. Using almost a standard 2:1 ratio (2 cups of water to 1 cup of grain), let the grain simmer until the water evaporates and add some pink salt and chopped fresh or dried herbs. I like to serve grains mixed with a salad, to get plenty of nutritious leafy greens combined with the carbohydrate energy; it makes me feel entertained and never bored of my salads. (For salad recipe ideas, check out the Recipe section, page 177.)

DAIRY PRODUCTS
milk, yoghurt, cheese

Cow milk is receiving a bad reputation due to how cows are treated, which consequently affects the quality of the milk, making it full of hormones, antibiotics, and not enough nutrition. Buying supermarket milk, which most of the time is pasteurized, can lead to increased inflammation in the body, a trigger for many health concerns. A 2011 study showed how cow milk can stimulate the growth of prostate cancer cells, and soya milk can stimulate the growth of breast cancer cells, whereas almond milk suppressed the growth of cancer cells by 30 percent.[26] There is a general thought that many of us are lactose intolerant, but most of the time it's simply that we have difficulty digesting the lactose in pasteurised milk. Unpasteurised, raw, organic milk from happy healthy cows is okay to drink if you like the taste and if you aren't sensitive to lactose. I once had a client whose son, aged six, had severe skin rashes on his face and back of the arms. After many doctor and dermatologist visits, they still had no solution to help the poor boy. I asked one question: How often does he drink milk? The answer was: Every day before bed. I recommended eliminating cow milk completely from his diet and applying coconut oil to his skin. After two weeks, the rashes calmed down, and after two more weeks, they were completely gone.

A popular myth exists in the dairy industry that Greek yoghurt is the healthier option. Unfortunately, it isn't so; Greek-style yoghurt doesn't differ at all from other conventionally made yoghurts. To claim that a product is genuine Greek-style, the yoghurt needs to go through the traditional process of straining the liquid whey, which removes some of the lactose sugar, salt, and water, making it quite thick. That's why this type of yoghurt may have more protein and less sugar and carbs. However, the FDA doesn't regulate the term "Greek-style", which gives many brands the freedom to add a thickening agent to the yoghurt, avoiding the traditional, more costly ways of thickening. And to top it all, the process of making the yoghurt includes pasteurisation, during which a high level of nutrition that dairy has to offer is destroyed. Without even realising it, frequent intake of Greek-style yoghurt could be the reason for your acne, skin flare-ups, hormonal trouble, and weight gain.

Cheese addiction is very common and is okay, providing you choose the right type of cheese. Processed, pasteurised, low-fat, sweetened cheeses are a bad choice for our health due to the fact that they come from unhealthy, hormone-injected cows; are full of sugar; and have no fat. I think that explains it all. For alternatives, read further!

HEALTHY DAIRY ALTERNATIVES
nut milks, raw full-fat yoghurt, kefir, healthy cheese options

Any type of nut milk—coconut, almond, cashew, walnut—has nutritional benefits, especially when it's homemade. In the section on kitchen equipment (page 75), you can read about a nut milk machine you can invest in, in order to have fresh homemade milk every day! Coconut milk is known for its lauric acid content, which helps you fight viruses and infections,[27] whereas almond milk has anti-inflammatory and antioxidant properties.[28] Rice milk may seem like a good option; however, it can be loaded with arsenic, as discussed previously.

Fermented, raw, full-fat yoghurt is a better alternative. The fermentation allows the yoghurt to provide you with protective health-promoting gut bacteria, and the fat provides vitamins A and D. Raw yoghurt hasn't gone through the process of pasteurisation when most nutrients are destroyed.

Kefir, a lactose-free fermented probiotic drink full of bioactive compounds, can help you build a strong gut to prevent many diseases arising. These bioactive compounds help your body absorb calcium, preventing bone degeneration, and, coupled with the generous amounts of K2 vitamin in kefir, you're set for strong, healthy bones. Kefir boosts the immune system, assists in healing skin allergies, helps the gut fight off infections, and helps eliminate irritable bowel syndrome.[29] You can purchase organic kefir from your local store or learn how to make your own.

It is possible to be a healthy cheese addict, in balance, of course! So here are your healthy options: feta cheese, goat cheese, ricotta cheese, cottage cheese, and Pecorino Romano cheese. Choose the organic unpasteurised options for maximum nutrition and least hormone intervention. Feta cheese is a source of calcium, vitamin B2, B12, selenium, and phosphorous. Goat cheese increases the absorption of iron from other foods and boosts the bioavailability of calcium. Ricotta and cottage cheeses are a good source of fat, yet it isn't advisable to overconsume them. Pecorino Romano cheese is an excellent source of protein: In just 28 grams, there are 7 grams of protein. A platter of the listed healthy cheeses once in a while could be a great source of key nutrients.[30]

Reflections

	How often do you consume?	Are you willing to stop buying the unhealthy version?	Are you willing to switch to healthy alternative versions?
Vegetable oils			
Table salt			
Sugar			
Refined carbs			
White rice			
Dairy products			

The first step to spread awareness is to get to know the subject.

Emotional Favourites

We've learned about the staple foods of every household: oil, salt, sugar, flour, grains, and dairy. It's almost impossible to run your kitchen and meals without them. Now, we'll explore the foods frequently found in kitchens that are unnecessary for the body and carry no nutritional value, but that we still tend to turn to when we're bored, TV binging, emotionally upset, stressed out, or trying to calm down a child.

Item	Why unhealthy?	Healthy alternative
Processed frozen foods	Contain starch which keeps the frozen food fresh, however starch is actually a polymer of glucose, shooting up your blood sugar whenever you eat frozen foods. These foods are also rich in trans fats, which raise LDL, leading to heart problems. With too much sugar,or too much salt, frozen foods contain preservatives that are seen as carcinogenic substances.[31]	Fresh foods eaten raw or cooked at home

Item	Why unhealthy?	Healthy alternative
Processed meats & sausages	Contain sodium nitrate which can be very detrimental to health, increasing the risks of diabetes type 1,[32] impaired oxygen transport in the body,[33] cancer,[34] and Alzheimer's disease.[35]	Organic meat without added hormones and antibiotics: beef, chicken, lamb
Nutella	Contains palm oil, a lot of sugar, and more sugar. Causes hyperactivity in children and inability for prolonged focus and concentration.	Homemade cocoa spread Avocado-Cashew Spread (see page 189)
Flavoured yoghurts & milkshakes	High content of sugar is very harmful to the body, as well as lactose, which can cause unnecessary bloating, allergies, weight gain.	Natural full-fat yoghurts Use nut/oat/rice milk instead of cow milk; use raw cocoa powder and real fruits instead of syrups
Salty nuts	High intake of sodium leads to weight gain, increase in blood pressure, water retention, and dehydration.	Raw nuts & seeds

Item	Why unhealthy?	Healthy alternative
Soft & carbonated drinks	Flavoured soft and carbonated drinks contain huge amount of sugar, even when it says natural 100% fruit. When it's packaged, it most certainly has preservatives. In addition to sugar content, carbonated drinks are very acidic and lead to a speedier ageing process.	Fresh green juices (must have a vegetable inside, otherwise fruits only spike up the insulin) Fresh green smoothies Kombucha
Chips	Trans fats, preservatives, sugar, salt – why even bother our cells with it?	Homemade vegetable chips: kale chips, beetroot chips, sweet potato chips (see page 188)
Ice cream	Very easy emotional snacks for any sad or happy moment. However, take your time to read the ingredients of these things when you purchase, and look for the sugar content, salt, preservatives, MSG, and any other word you cannot pronounce.	Coconut yoghurt ice cream Frozen fruit
Chocolates & candy		80% or higher dark chocolate
Biscuits & cookies		Homemade cookies, muffins, brownies (see page 191)

The items in this table might be in your shopping cart, cupboards, or fridge just for that one cheat meal or special occasion. However, if you're used to buying these items regularly, then the chances are that you or the members of your house quite enjoy them, are almost addicted to them, and notice no health problems associated with these "foods". That's because of your emotional attachment to them.

When I started my journey of health, I was living with my parents. I realised how unhealthy the contents of our fridge were and was preaching to my parents to stop buying the foods that killed their health. They listened 80 percent of the time, but one item—ice cream—my dad bought every week and hid in the freezer behind my packs of organic frozen berries. He'd eat a scoop of it every night while he watched the news, because to not eat anything in front of the TV is almost impossible, right? What do you think I did when I found out? I started looking for ice cream alternatives. I bought an ice cream maker. I baked alternative healthy desserts. But as much as he appreciated all my efforts, I couldn't beat the taste of ice cream. Even though he experienced poor quality of sleep or even occasional evening bloating, he didn't stop indulging in his favourite "food". Apart from this cheat meal, what helps him keep his form are the daily 6 km morning walks, his morning green juices and green smoothies, healthy breakfast, balanced afternoon meal, and, of course, his positive character. It's very difficult for a person to change lifelong habits, but it's possible to introduce some healthy lifestyle improvements that have a chance to counteract any unhealthy habits. It may not be the long-term solution; however, it provides time and flexibility for the person to make their own conscious decisions rather than being told what to do.

Another example is my cousin, who was a sugar addict. He knew it, but the battle inside his head was too strong to fight, and he gave in to any temptation, especially when he was stressed, upset, or simply bored. It's truly difficult for someone to give up sweets, no matter the reason you give them. However, after he independently decided to do the five-week program from my book

Wake Up!, his outlook has been transformed. After the five weeks of clean eating and no sugar, he realised how sugar contributed tô his poor-quality sleep, chronic fatigue, inability to focus, mood swings, and just a general "blah" feeling. He still has moments when he's fighting the craving, and even moments when he does give in to the temptation, but the big difference between then and now is that he makes a conscious choice to either avoid it or eat it. It's no longer an emotional reaction when he gets lost in the indulgence, wanting more and more.

It's a matter of training that muscle, just as you would train your biceps, for example. Ten reps won't make a difference; you'll only start seeing definition after weeks and months of regular practice. So, referring back to the muscle that counteracts your cravings or unhealthy temptations, it takes time and practice. Sometimes you fail, and that's okay, but it only takes continuity and consistently questioning "do I need this?" for you to build up resistance. This applies to not only sugar addictions but also other unhealthy addictions such as alcohol, coffee, smoking, and so on.

When I go grocery shopping, I hardly ever go into the middle aisles of the supermarket, except to buy some organic grains, raw apple cider vinegar, frozen organic berries, and organic sustainable cleaning products. I don't buy the foods in the previous table, and everyone who visits me is aware of my attitude toward these things. My guests bring me fruits, selections of nuts, or even dark chocolate. I was never shy about explaining the detrimental aspects of these foods for our body and how I wouldn't choose to have them in my "temple"—my home. And this decision allows me to have cheat meals once in a while when I'm out dining, socialising, or travelling, absolutely guilt free. Because I know that when I'm at home—and I prefer to eat at home 80 percent of the week—my body enjoys natural, highly nutritious, delicious foods.

Another small but relevant detail about my eating habits: I'm not emotionally attached to food. When I'm stressed or upset, I write. I write it all out in my journal; it lifts a lot of pressure from my shoulders and clears my mind to take conscious steps to mitigating a particular situation.

A very useful quick practice I introduce to my clients to help them through an overwhelm of emotions is the Emotional Freedom Technique (EFT). EFT focuses on meridian spots where the energy of the body flows through. By tapping on these spots, it is believed that we restore the energy balance, which relieves the body of negative physical or emotional blockages.

When you feel your emotions rising and the only way you've ever known to suppress it is through food, alcohol, or drugs . . . give tapping a try. Take a look at the diagram and lightly tap those points of your body while repeating the following sentence as you tap each point.

"Even though I feel {emotion}, I fully and deeply love and accept myself."

Perform three rounds of this, then take a deep inhale and exhale and note how you feel. Tapping will most certainly shift something.

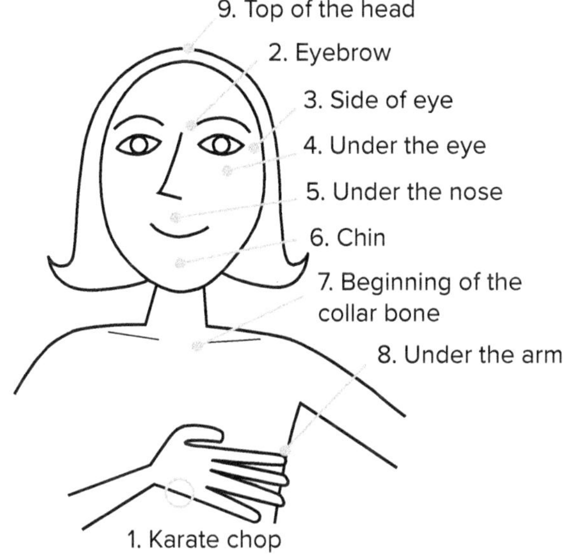

You can also crowd out unhealthy cravings with healthy food alternatives, interesting activities, and a healthy home environment, which this book is all about! Keep questioning, "Do I need this?" "Is this an emotional choice or is it a conscious decision to eat this food?" Even if, after questioning, you still go ahead and indulge in your unhealthy craving, that's also okay. At least you asked yourself, and after some time of practicing and questioning, you'll actually react. Believe me.

Reflections

How often do you and your family consume the unhealthy foods listed in the table (page 49)?

What do you think is your main trigger for emotional eating? How can you support yourself when the trigger shows up again?

How do you feel about the healthy alternatives provided to you?

Importance of Organic Food

"Foods that we eat are probably
the main pathway to pesticide exposure"
Environmental Health Perspectives, 2008

We're all seeing and experiencing the craze for organic products, from organic vegetables to organic chicken to organic nuts to organic shampoos and organic toilet cleaners. When it's organic, then naturally it's better and, of course, more expensive. Many of us see the "organic" label as a marketing tool, which is far from the truth, and I'm happy to have the chance here to explain why.

The word "organic" means something that grows without any interference. So, if an apple tree can grow without being sprayed with pesticides and herbicides, and chickens are allowed to roam around without being injected with hormones and antibiotics, then these products are considered natural and clean (i.e., organic). Not long ago, everything that our great-grandparents grew up on was natural and clean, and it was only in the 1940s that Swiss chemist Paul Muller discovered the first synthetic pesticide, called "dichlorodiphenyltrichloroethane", or DDT, which was able to kill the pests that were destroying the farming industry.[36] Muller was awarded a Noble Prize for his discovery and we were awarded a future full of disease outbreaks, as suddenly we went from eating food to eating chemicals.

The chemicals that are sprayed on our food crops kill the brains of the insects, and it's only a matter of time that this consistent intake of chemicals will bring our brains and bodies to a complete stop, too. The sad truth is that when we think we're shopping for food, we're not; we're shopping for chemicalized products that have been artificially grown. How can our body cells thrive and regenerate on these chemicals?

Sometimes, it may seem that our world has turned against us, a world that would rather feed us chemicals to create and treat disease, rather than feed us natural foods in order to prevent disease.

This book is your trigger to find local organic foods in your area and to do your calculations. It's best not to buy organic in the supermarkets but directly from the farms, so you can help them be sustainable. You'll spend a little more money on your groceries, but the results of clean eating will be so obvious on your health, on your energy, on your focus, and even on your mood, that it will all be worth it. Don't be frightened by the word organic. What I would be frightened of are the pesticides that are being sprayed left, right, and centre.

If purchasing organic isn't accessible to you, the next best alternative is to soak your fruits and vegetables in a water and apple cider vinegar mix (1 cup water to 3 tablespoons of apple cider vinegar). This mix will remove some of the pesticides from your foods. Or you can just remove the peels of the fruits and vegetables whenever possible. The Environmental Working Group provides a "dirty dozen" list, and it is always best to purchase these items organic.[37]

DIRTY DOZEN

Strawberries	Peaches	Cherries	Bell peppers
Apples	Celery	Spinach	Cherry tomatoes
Nectarines	Grapes	Tomatoes	Cucumbers

I buy all my foods organic, organic products for my skin and hair, and "green" organic cleaning products for the house. I have visited the farm that grows various foods that I buy, and I'm certain of the quality and their intentions. You could do that, too! I strongly hope that you'll take this message to heart and will look for the best possible options for yourself.

Reflections

What do you believe are your barriers to switching to organic foods? How could you start the process of buying more organic?

THE BATHROOM

Your skin is an organ, the largest and the heaviest in your body, and is made up of numerous nerves, glands, and cell layers that all play a crucial role in various functions of the body. Skin is also your protective shield that can withstand certain temperatures and toxic chemicals. Moreover, it secretes antibacterial compounds that protect you from infection and bacteria from the external environment. Now, imagine moisturising your liver, which is also an organ, with creams that are full of chemicals, or spraying your heart with expensive French perfume, or applying deodorant to your kidneys. Why would you imagine doing such things? Well, simply because you regularly wash your body with scented shower gel, use antibacterial soap for your hands, moisturise your skin with chemical-loaded creams, spray yourself with perfume, and much more. Anything that's applied to the skin gets absorbed immediately into the rest of the body. Although skin is the largest and heaviest organ, it's also the thinnest—less than one-tenth of an inch protects your internal organs from potential toxins. Day after day, the average woman is exposed to over 500 chemicals in her daily regimen, which adds up to tens of thousands of chemicals over her lifetime entering her blood, lymph system, and organs, disrupting her immune system, hormonal system, and every other system in her body.

As a teenager, I used to love to buy a brand of deliciously scented shower gels. After every shower, my skin would be as dry and wrinkled as a raisin. My solution? Smother my body with another "ready to eat" scented moisturiser. I suffered from severe itching on my legs and dry skin during the day and had to constantly apply lots of cream to reduce the dryness. I also had lots of white pimples on the backs of my arms. Never did I associate the products I was using with the dryness or the itching. I also used to own five or six different perfumes at a time and wouldn't leave the house without adding that "personal" touch to my attire. Applying nail polish to my fingernails and toenails every two weeks was equal to brushing my teeth with toothpaste loaded with chemicals. I also had a very weak immune system and was sick every second month of the year.

What we put on our skin is a serious matter, and I invite you to educate yourself more about it so you can adopt improvements relevant to you and also be an example to others. First, let's dissect what chemicals are hiding in our day-to-day products sitting in our bathrooms and why they're dangerous for our health.

Product	Chemicals	Why harmful?
Anti-bacterial soap	Triclosan[1]	Antibiotic resistance; endocrine disruption; harmful to environment
Shower gel	Triclosan, Parabens, SLS, Dioxane, Propylene glycol, DEA Perfume, Toluene[2]	Carcinogenic substances; endocrine disruption; toxic to brain, nervous system, liver, kidneys; dries out the skin
Shampoo / Conditioner		

Product	Chemicals	Why harmful?
Toothpaste	Fluoride, Triclosan, SLS, Parabens, Carrageenan, Propylene glycol, DEA, Microbeads[3]	Carcinogenic substances; neurological dysfunction; endocrine disruption; thyroid dysfunction; intestinal inflammation; harmful to environment
Body moisturiser Face cream	Mineral oil and many other chemicals[4]	Mineral oil is a derivative from petroleum – carcinogenic; inhibits skin's natural respiratory process, leading to pimples and blackheads
Deodorant / Antiperspirant	Aluminium, Parabens, Phthalates, Triclosan, Fragrances[5]	Breast cancer; hormonal imbalances; thyroid dysfunction
Perfumes	Fragrance (have the right not to expose which ingredients are used)[6]	Synthetic chemicals linked to cancer; reproductive toxicity; allergies; and more
Nail polish	DBP, Toluene (from petroleum), Formaldehyde[7]	Carcinogenic substances; anemia; lower blood count; liver or kidney damage; harmful to fetus (pregnancy)

Product	Chemicals	Why harmful?
Hair dye	Coal tar, Formaldehyde, Eugenol, DMDM Hydantoin, Para-phenylenediamine, Tetrahydro-6-nitroquinoxaline[8]	Carcinogenic substances; immunotoxic; developmental and reproductive toxicity; neurotoxicity; allergies
Make up	Lead, Beryllium, Thallium, Cadmium, Arsenic[9]	Reproductive disorders; neurological problems; mood swings; memory loss; muscle and joint loss; headaches; hair loss; endocrine disruptors
Shaving cream	Mineral oil (same as body and face lotions)	Mineral oil is a derivative from petroleum – carcinogenic; inhibits skin's natural respiratory process, leading to pimples and blackheads
Sun protection (commercial SPF lotions)	Oxybenzone, Fragrances, Retinyl Palmitate[10]	Endocrine disruptor; decreased sperm count; endometriosis in women

I want you to be able to walk into your bathroom, look at every single product and be 100 percent certain that these products only nourish your body and soften and replenish your skin with essential vitamins for longevity and elasticity. My healthy sustainable alternatives for every possible product that you may need for self-care are laid out in the table on page 66. These are without harmful side effects for you, without cruel animal testing, and are simple products designed by Mother Nature for us to use.

Coconut oil is very moisturising, antibacterial, antifungal, anti-inflammatory, and a powerful source of antioxidants, which fight the free radicals we're exposed to daily. However, it may clog the skin on your face and result in breakouts, so when you do use it for makeup removal, make sure to wash or cleanse your face thoroughly afterward to get rid of any oily residue.

In my own bathroom, I have natural soaps for body, hair, and hands; organic rosehip, grapeseed, and sweet almond oils for my body and face; and organic natural charcoal-based toothpaste. The number of plastic bottles purchased has drastically decreased since I don't buy fancy shower gels or shampoos anymore, and all my oils come in glass jars. Not only does my body feel good being nourished with all the vitamins and minerals, but I also feel I'm positively contributing to the future of our environment.

It can take a little time to get used to using natural products. Maybe they don't have that scrumptious luxurious smell when you put them on, but here's a tip: Whatever smells too good has had chemicals and preservatives added to enhance the aromas.

When you strive to be healthy, what you put on the outside of your body is equally as important as what you put inside your body. I would like you to realise that your skin health and body care is literally in your hands. Just because harmful ingredients are sold in the market doesn't mean they're safe to use; moreover, they damage your current health and the health of our environment.

Toxic Product	Healthy Alternative
Antibacterial soap	Natural soaps e.g., olive oil soap
Shower gel	Natural soaps
Shampoo / Conditioner	Natural soaps, toxin-free shampoos
Toothpaste	Fluoride-free toothpaste Charcoal-based toothpaste
Body moisturiser	Natural oils: coconut oil, sesame oil, shea butter
Body scrub / Face scrub	Coconut oil w/Epsom salts Ground coffee w/olive oil Ground oat flakes with yoghurt
Face cream	Natural oils like jojoba or grapeseed oil, natural ingredients-based facial creams, natural serums with vitamins A and E
Deodorant	Dry natural soap, baking soda w/water, toxic-free deodorant
Perfumes	Natural fragrances from essential oils
Nail polish	Toxin-free nail polish
Hair dye	Toxin-free hair dye / henna
Make up	Natural ingredients-based make up

Toxic Product	Healthy Alternative
Make up remover	Coconut oil
Shaving cream	Coconut oil Aloe vera gel
Sun protection	Coconut oil / almond oil / toxin-free SPF

Reflections

Do you and your family purchase and use commercial skin-body care products? Specify which ones. Are you ready to switch to the alternatives mentioned? What do you think would be your obstacles to making the change?

CLEAN YOUR HOME WITH CLEAN PRODUCTS

t's very hard to believe that your home could be the source of indoor pollution and could, consequently, lead to asthma, lung degeneration, skin problems, and hormonal imbalances. In a recent study by the World Health Organisation, 92 percent of the global population is inhaling polluted air from transportation vehicles, coal-powered factories, industrial activities, and burning of household fuel.[1] We try to get away from these obvious culprits and spend more time in natural habitats or building our homes farther away from the cities. However, polluted air can be still be in your bedrooms, bathrooms, and living room. A study recently published by the *American Journal of Respiratory and Critical Care Medicine* showcases that fine particulate air pollution could be released while you're cleaning your home.[2]

How did our grandmothers or their mothers clean their house? I don't believe they had powerful fragrant detergents to kill all bacteria. I asked my grandmother once what people used to clean their homes when she was young back in the 1930s, and the answer was simple: water, soap, and vinegar. Since the 1950s, the market has been infiltrated by a huge selection of toxic cleaning products to give us the quickest, most fragrant way to clean the dirtiest of places. And now I wonder if there's any connection between us getting sicker and the world getting more chemicalised?

"Once-weekly use of cleaning products for 20 years may be equivalent to smoking 20 cigarettes a day for 10 to 20 years." This result from a research study carried out in Norway[3] signifies how the chemicals in these cleaning products irritate and damage the mucus membrane lining of the lungs, as they evaporate into the air when used or even during storage. Have you ever noticed that the cleaning product aisle in the supermarket smells pretty fragrant? This is a sign that volatile organic compounds (VOCs) are being released into the air. When inhaled by us, dependent on frequency and concentration, they may cause serious damage to our health. Avoid those aisles and avoid those products!

The short-term impact on your health may result in asthma; nose, eye, and throat irritation; headaches; and fatigue, whereas the long-term impact, although not thoroughly researched, could lead to cancer or reduced lung function.

The air in your home may be two to five times more polluted than the air outside, according to the Environmental Protection Agency, an astonishing fact that could be the invisible source of so many of our troubles. My question now is why these products are still widely available for purchase. Your next question might be: How can I make smart choices for my home?

HEALTHY ALTERNATIVES FOR CLEANING PRODUCTS

Certified organic cleaning products, such as toilet cleaner, glass and window cleaner, dishwasher liquid, floor cleaner, surface cleaner, etc., are available. All these products have plant-based ingredients, are vegan (no animal testing), contain no chemicals, are biodegradable, and reduce chemical waste and pollution. As well as looking after the quality of the air in your home, by buying organic cleaning products, you will also contribute positively to the environment and Mother Earth.

As an alternative to purchasing products, here is a useful table on how you can clean your home using the basics: water, white vinegar, natural soap, castile soap, lemon, and coconut oil. Not only will you save money, you'll also buy far fewer plastic bottles.

Dishwasher detergent	Mix equal parts castile soap and water. Store the mixture in a jar easily accessible to you during dishwashing or adding to the dishwasher machine.
Antibacterial solution (toilet seat, toilet bowl)	Mix 2 cups water with 3 tablespoons castile soap and 20–30 drops tea tree oil. Store in a spray bottle.
Bathtub &shower cleaning paste	Mix 2 tablespoons baking soda with 2 teaspoons castile soap to create a paste. Scrub on the area and wash off with water.
Glass & window cleaner	Mix 2 cups water with ½ cup white vinegar and ¼ cup rubbing alcohol concentration (70%). Add a few drops of favourite essential oil. Put in a spray bottle.

Multisurface floor cleaner	Mix 2 tablespoons castile soap into a bucket of hot water. Add a few drops of your favourite essential oil. Mop the floor. Add clean hot water to the bucket, without soap, and clean the floor again.
Scented all-purpose cleaner	Mix 1 cup water with 1 cup white vinegar, add rosemary sprigs and lemon peel. Allow it to settle for a week; afterwards, use it to clean anything you need (carpet stains, kitchen counter top, etc.)

Your laundry room is perhaps the most toxic room in the house, yet we would never normally associate any of our health problems with the washing powder that we use or the comforting "rose" smell from our clothes. The chemicals in laundry detergent can produce negative health effects ranging from throat, eye, and skin irritation to being carcinogenic.[4]

Most laundry product manufacturers aren't required to list all the ingredients in their products, and when they mention "fragrance", that word alone could encompass hundreds of chemicals, some of which are hazardous. Even when advertised as "fragrance free", they could still contain petrochemicals to trick you into the freshness and pleasant smell. Liquid clothes softeners contain chemicals that never leave the clothes—to provide that softness—and therefore come into contact with your skin. In addition to being dangerous for your well-being, the chemicals in laundry products get released into the water supply, and because they decompose very slowly or hardly at all, they contaminate the environment and kill marine life.

This is enough information for us to turn to alternatives! You could be either buying organic, chemical-free, plant-based detergents, which can be expensive, or you could make your own! I've been using this recipe for a while now.

16 cups baking soda
12 cups washing soda (sodium carbonate, easily found in a supermarket)
8 cups grated castile soap
3 tablespoons essential oil, for natural fragrance (e.g., lavender, lemon, orange, grapefruit)

Combine everything, whisk, and keep in an airtight jar. You can use ⅛ cup for a 4-kilogram load. You can pre-treat any stains on clothing with a paste of baking soda, washing soda, and water. If you want to give your washing machine a "cleanse", run a cleaning cycle with just white vinegar and hot water. This will get rid of any bacteria, grease, or scum that has accumulated in your machine over time.

You may now have a lot of questions in your head. Good. That's my plan. I want us to wake up from the unconscious lifestyle that we've been living, a lifestyle that's harmful to us, our children, and Mother Nature. It's time to wake up to the truth that you have given your whole human body over to other entities to manage. Take your power back, question every single ingredient, and, even better, turn to Mother Nature and ask: What would you do?

Reflections

How often do you and your family members use toxic cleaning products and detergents in your house? How do you feel about the information in this chapter? Are you ready to turn to environmentally healthy alternatives?

WAYS TO ENHANCE YOUR HOME

KITCHEN EQUIPMENT

Without getting into too much science and complexity, do you think food with torn and deformed molecules is something our great-grandparents would consider normal? Nutritious? Life extending? Microwave ovens were introduced to the world forty years ago, but only recently have there been in-depth, open, but still not enough studies about the various ways a microwave can inflict damage on our health. Don't get me wrong; I used to microwave my daily lunch at work and eat my "healthy meal" with so much pride, to only feel bloated afterward. I never realised that my broccoli and carrots had lost all their nutrients in the microwave and were now deformed chemical compounds. According to a 1991 study by Dr Hertel, a Swiss scientist, because of microwaving, the deformed food molecules contain radiolytic compounds, which are suggested to also have carcinogenic potential. If that's the case, why are these "convenient" food machines even sold? According to the industry, there isn't enough compelling evidence that microwaves can cause such harm. How about the fact that microwave ovens operate on a frequency similar to a 4G cellular network?[1] So as you stand there waiting for your meal to heat up, you're exposed to radiation densities thousands of times higher than your mobile phone gives off. This type of radiation waves can cause immediate and dramatic changes to your heart rate and heart rate variability. Does this sound sensible to you? Microwaving in plastic Tupperware or bags exposes you to toxic chemicals such as BPA and phthalates (I can't even pronounce the latter!). If this information isn't enough for you to make the decision to get rid of your microwave, I urge you to study this topic further, and I sincerely hope you'll make the right choice to benefit yourself and your loved ones.

"Microwaving breast milk destroys the essential disease-fighting agents that offer protection for the baby. On the contrary it was found that microwaving fosters the growth of more potentially hazardous pathogens" – from the 1992 study "Effects of microwave radiation on anti-infective factors in human milk."[2]

The microwave oven is the first and perhaps only item of kitchen equipment that I would label hazardous.

Here is a list of kitchen equipment I recommend investing in, and each one can be used to enhance and ease your new healthy lifestyle.

ITEM	USAGE
Blender	Make smoothies, soups
Juicer	Make fresh juice
Food processor	Chop vegetables, slice nuts, seeds, mix dough, etc
Steamer	Steam vegetables, chicken, fish

ITEM	USAGE
Pressure cooker	Quickly cook rice and beans
Nut milk machine	Make homemade milk
Pasta machine	Thin homemade pasta
Grain mill	Grind grain into flour for baking bread
Bread machine	Bake homemade bread
Dehydrator	Make chips

I'm not suggesting that you have to buy all this equipment at once; you may even have some already. I would suggest that you start using the items you have regularly so you get used to it, like your juicer or blender. After a few months, you might invest in a nut milk machine, use it, get familiar with it, and after a few more months, purchase another item. My advice is to really study each machine and understand whether it can be of use and complement your current busy lifestyle.

NATURE AT HOME

I'm a plant-crazy person! I never really studied them or how to look after them, never really had any plants during my childhood, but I do clearly remember my grandmother and her love for nature and animals. She was a biologist and had a small garden that she took great care of. She spent hours in the garden, always fed the birds, and kept food aside for street dogs and cats. I miss her very much and am so grateful for the small lessons that she taught me in my early years of life. I feel that I've inherited her love and empathy for plants and animals. I talk to my plants and thank them for their beauty. I feed the birds and have rescued little ones from hungry crows. I have two rescue dogs and a rescue cat at home and have never felt so close to nature, although I live in a very unnatural place—Dubai!

Having a natural environment at home with house plants not only benefits you spiritually and psychologically but is also one of the most affordable ways to reduce indoor pollution by purifying the air, cleansing the odours, absorbing various toxins, and even providing humidity for the home. In the previous section about using "green" cleaning products, we talked about how our indoor pollution can be several times worse than outside air pollution due to off-gassing furniture, paint, carpeting and other flooring, building materials, furniture fabrics, printers, cleaning products, air fresheners, candles, acetone, nail polish, perfume, and even dry-cleaned clothes. It's frightening to think of the amount of chemicals and toxins we breathe in daily in our homes! But no need to panic; Mother Nature has given us a solution.

In 2006, Vadoud Niri, a chemist from the State University of New York, presented to the American Chemical Society his team's findings on how houseplants effectively reduce indoor air pollution. It is a very interesting study, well worth looking into, that identified which plants removed exactly which chemical toxins, at what rate, and how much of these air toxins were eventually removed from the air. They listed twelve plants that do the job the best.

Bromeliad	Purifies the air by 90 percent from the benzene emitted from paint, furniture wax, detergent, and glue.
Dracena	Absorbs 90 percent of the acetone released from household cleaners and nail polish removers. So, if you aren't ready yet to switch to "green" household cleaning products, adopt a few Dracaena to keep your mind at peace!
Spider plant	Absorbs up to 90 percent of formaldehyde and carbon monoxide from smoking, and P-xylene from plastics. I have a few scattered around the house, although we have a nonsmoking family, but I admire the spider plant for fighting the plastic outgassing chemicals!
Jade plant	Very good at absorbing toluene, a gas emitted from paint, lacquers, gasoline, and kerosene. A perfect plant for beauty salons!
Ferns	Able to provide humidity. Especially good if you live in an environment where the air can get a little dry.
Peace lily	My favourite little helper, because it absorbs electromagnetic radiation from devices and humidifies the air. In my home, I keep one next to the Wi-Fi box and one next to the computer.
English ivy	A beautiful houseplant with the power to remove the toxins from cigarette smoking and even assist people suffering from asthma by cleansing the air.
Ficus	Removes odours and decreases the amount of toxic substances in the air of your home or office.

Snake plant	Removes benzene and formaldehyde. It is best kept in the bedroom as it increases the oxygen supply in the room at night.
Philoden-dron	Efficiently detoxifies formaldehyde.
Bamboo palm (reed palm)	Absorbs the formaldehyde off-gassing from furniture. If you have bought a new piece of furniture it would be good to place a few of these plants around it.

It is very important to note that if you're allergic or sensitive to mould, keeping plants at home may aggravate your sensitivity due to mould settling on the soil and leaves. However, there is a way to combat this: Clean the leaves with a wet paper towel, remove the top part of the soil where the mould is visible, replace it with fresh potting soil, and make sure your pot has good drainage.

Bear in mind that many of the listed plants are poisonous to dogs and cats when ingested. Many of my houseplants are out of reach for my dogs, but, even so, they know they are not allowed to hurt my green "babies". Aside from the listed plants, of course, you can have many others. I enjoy keeping mint, basil, and thyme, as I often use them in salads and dressings. I also have an aloe vera plant, and, once a week, I use the aloe vera gel on my face or hair. Plants are our friends and have a beautiful ability to complement our mental well-being and further enhance our health.

When potting plants, please consider the type of pot that you use. Plastic pots, which are very common, also give off toxins that may also leak into the soil of your plants, affecting their growth and health. It's ironic to consider that you keep a plant in order to cleanse the air, but keeping it in a plastic pot counteracts the initial intention. Clay or ceramic pots with good drainage will keep your plants happy and provide an attractive touch to your home.

A further tip is, whether you're an advanced gardener or a beginner, consider acquiring a mobile application called Parrot Power Flower and purchasing a thermometer that's connected to the app. You can insert the thermometer into the plant pot, and in the app you'll read exactly what your plant needs: more or less water, more sunlight, fertilizer, etc. What I've learned from my experience with plants is that I don't need to be an expert, but I do need to give them love. They give me so much more than I could ever offer in return, but I know my attention, care, love, a bit of water, and sun is all they really want.

Another way of connecting with nature is to provide a feeding plate or bowl for birds on your balcony, window shelf, or garden. It will take a few days, maybe a couple of weeks, for the birds to realise that it's safe to come and eat, but once one comes, it will tell all its friends, and you'll hear constant tweeting outside your window, bringing more life and positive vibes to your home. I like to feed the birds hulled millet. That way, I know they're getting a good source of protein and minerals and good quality carbohydrates rather than spiking up their sugar levels with breadcrumbs.

Bringing nature into your home isn't so difficult after all.

PERSONALISING YOUR HOME SCENT

Natural essential oils can help us with various health concerns ranging from asthma to ADHD.[3] There are hundreds of varieties: lavender, ylang ylang, frankincense, oregano, tea tree, and so on, and each one has numerous benefits. Without getting into too many details, I encourage you to have an inviting home scent that will trigger positive vibes and good energy, besides the health benefits, of course. Below, you'll find some ways you can create an inviting aroma in your home. I recommend sticking to one method, finding your favourite smell, and making that the trademark of your home. That way, when family and friends enter your home, they will immediately feel a sense of familiarity, trust, and absolute relaxation. You can try out the recipes I provide or create your own, but, most importantly, find the scent that makes your whole being fill with serenity and joy.

Essential oil diffuser	An ultrasonic aromatherapy diffuser or a nebulizing diffuser is the easiest way to give your home the scent and happy vibes you want. Decide which machine suits you best, pick your oils for each mood, and enjoy the scents for hours.
Incense	It is very important to invest in high-quality natural incense, which is also an easy way to create a sense of mystique in your home.
Burning candles	Don't burn commercial scented candles, as they release petroleum-based chemicals into the air and many other toxic substances that can heavily contribute to your indoor pollution.[4] Beeswax candles can actually help people with various allergies, asthma, and hay fever by releasing negative ions. They're pricier, but I would rather live without candles than breathe in toxins. What do you think?
Dried herbs with a candle	Take any dried herb of preference, such as lavender, cinnamon, or rosemary, crush them in a bowl, and light a small candle in the middle. It creates a delicate aroma that may be best placed in the bathroom or next to your bed.

Simmering spices	This is a wonderful way to create a scent in your kitchen, especially to eliminate a cooking smell; however, I wouldn't recommend it all the time, as your gas/electricity consumption would increase. Put various spices into a pot of water, bring it to a boil, then simmer for as long as you like, topping up with water. Try this recipe: cinnamon sticks, apple peels, orange rinds, whole cloves. You can mix and match dry herbs with citrus fruits, and maybe a few drops of vanilla.
Spray bottle with essential oils	For 1 tablespoon of water, add 10 drops of essential oil. Fill a small spray bottle and use it anytime during the day.

The aroma scent of my home . . . I won't tell you, because it's a trademark recipe, but one thing you can be sure of, the aroma represents my whole being, lots of energy, and smiles! I have a scent for each room in my house; it's very fun and makes you smile whenever you walk into the space.

REDUCE ELECTROMAGNETIC FREQUENCY (EMF) EXPOSURE

"May 2011, the International Agency on Cancer Research, one of the arms of World Health Organisation, classified radiofrequency EMF—radiation from cellphones—a class 2B carcinogen, meaning it's possibly carcinogenic to humans."

Your mobile phone, laptop, tablet, Wi-Fi router, TV, microwave, baby monitors, and Bluetooth devices such as watches, keyboards, and computer mice all emit a certain degree of radiation. This wouldn't be a cause for concern if this exposure didn't possibly lead to negative health effects. EMFs activate the voltage-gated calcium channels (VGCCs) in the outer membrane of the cell, the plasma membrane that surrounds all our cells.[5] As the VGCCs are activated, they open and allow calcium ions into the cells. Excess calcium ions cause defects at a mitochondrial level, setting our body up for a chronic disease.

Furthermore, excessive calcium leads to a chemical chain reaction that contributes to the release of the most dangerous free radicals for a human. All of this sounds very technical and science-orientated, but all you really need to understood is that it isn't a good idea to activate the VGCCs in your body for whatever reason, especially the areas that are most VGCC-dense—such as the brain, the pacemaker in the heart, male testes—and therefore more prone to experience damage. Excessive calcium ions, oxidative stress, and low-frequency radiation exposure can be linked to health issues such as cardiac arrhythmias, anxiety, depression, autism, Alzheimer's, infertility, and even cancer.[6]

I'm not saying you should move to a wooden house deep in the forest. What I do sincerely hope is that you use this information for your benefit and equip yourself with the knowledge and tools so you can protect yourself from all angles. There's very little we can do to affect the electronics industry or even to decrease EMF exposure in our office, but we can certainly create a safe environment in our home. Below, you'll find some practical ways to decrease your EMF exposure and protect your cells from deforming unnecessarily.

- Unplug your Wi-Fi router and TV at night. It's an unnecessary exposure to the magnetic fields when your body is in high need of rest and repair. I had clients who used to have two to three Wi-Fi routers around the house, and one of them would be in their bedroom next to the TV that they watch right as they fall asleep. Exposure alert! And it would be the same people who would complain about light sleep and fatigue during the day, for which, of course, they would take too many cups of coffee, which, in turn, would raise the acidity in their body (leading to migraines, heartburn, ulcers, allergies, skin problems) and eventually increasing their body inflammation (leading to digestive issues, joint pain, chronic fatigue) and so on. Of course, this isn't to say your Wi-Fi box has the sole responsibility for how you feel today, but eliminating this possible contributor would be a good idea.

- Talk on the phone only with headphones. Especially if you do tend to talk on your mobile phone a lot, invest in a pair of headphones (not wireless!) and get into the habit of always using it.
- Your house phone shouldn't be wireless. Now we tend to talk more often and longer on the house phone, and we love that we can move around whilst keeping up the conversation. I remember this being such a miracle as a child when my parents brought a wireless phone home. I would call my friend, move around the house, and ask "Can you still hear me? And now? What about now? What if I go into the bathroom, can you still hear me?" And the crisp and clear connection had me wondering at this magic, not realising that this was the beginning of our "human destruction".
- Put your mobile phone on airplane mode. "But I use it as my alarm!" you may say. Oh, come on, what did your grandmother use as an alarm? I bet she didn't even have to use it because she would fall asleep reading her book, enjoy her deep quality sleep unaffected by magnetic fields, and wake up refreshed to eat her healthy natural breakfast. First things first: A traditional alarm clock will wake you up.

Putting your phone on airplane mode while you sleep, or just whenever you don't require it, is a good idea to limit the exposure of very high-frequency magnetic fields. Why do you think cabin crew on planes ask everyone to switch off their phones during the flight? A question many of us may not have thought about . . . What does your small device have or emit that may affect the flight of a huge airplane?

- Hardwire the internet to your laptop. I work on my laptop a lot, especially when I attend to my clients overseas through video calls, and in order to protect myself from EMF exposure, the internet on my laptop is hardwired rather than through an invisible Wi-Fi connection. Of course, I'm only able to do this when I work at home; it's much more difficult to apply when working from cafes.
- Avoid using a wireless keyboard, mouse, and printer. As convenient as these tools may be, it's an unnecessary radiation exposure due to their Bluetooth connections.
- Limit your use of gadgets that are Bluetooth connected to your phone, for the same reasons previously mentioned.
- Avoid placing your laptop on your lap whilst connected to the Wi-Fi. Use a mobile phone pouch that's shielded on one side. This decreases the exposure to a small extent when you carry the phone in your pocket with the shielded side against your body.

Here's my personal routine with my mobile phone and Wi-Fi exposure: I turn off the Wi-Fi box before sleep and turn it back on as we're ready to start the day. I put my mobile phone on airplane mode at 9 p.m. and purposefully forget it in a completely different room. I go against the habit of "scrolling down" on my phone before sleep and even in the morning, and only turn it back on when I'm done with my self-care routine and have already walked the dogs. I talk only through a headset and have no gadgets connected to my phone, except the Parrot Flower Power that I use occasionally. My TV is unplugged most of the time, unless I want to watch it, which does happen on a rare occasion!

It may seem pretty difficult to get your head around this. You may be wondering why there's no public warning on these products and devices. Trust me, I keep asking the same thing, only to realise that if I don't take control of my own lifestyle and health and make my own conscious choices, I'll be doomed to a physical and mental catastrophe. I hope I've triggered questions in your head, questions that will eventually lead to your own decisions to live your life without external influence.

SUSTAINABLE HOME

A sustainable home means a home that creates a fruitful future for generations to come. Whether it's for the children in your home or for the people outside, you're setting an example that will have a ripple effect into the future.

One of the main ways our environment is being hurt is through the use of plastic and its inability to degrade safely and rapidly.

Plastic was created in 1907, when scientists learned to break down crude oil to form polymers (i.e., plastic that can form any shape desired). It was an absolute brilliant discovery back then, which even gave a push to progress in many industries around the world, yet today plastic is considered to be the number one mass killer for the environment and its inhabitants, humans and animals alike. The main reason is because industries started using plastic for products that end up in the trash. That wouldn't be a problem if plastic didn't take from five hundred to a thousand years to degrade. According to an extensive study by the

UN Environment Programme, 40 percent of plastic produced is used for packaging alone. Since 1907, 8.3 billion metric tonnes of plastic were produced, 335 million metric tonnes in 2016 alone. Since 1907, more than 6.3 billion metric tonnes of plastic have become waste, 9 percent of which was recycled, 12 percent burnt (imagine the air pollution!) and 79 percent is lying around the world somewhere.[7] Most of it, around 13 million tonnes, ends up in the ocean every single year. And the number will increase as the world population rises. This is such a huge number that it could outweigh the amount of fish by 2050.

The sea world is suffering and, in 2018, a dead whale off the coast of Spain was found to have eaten 32 kg of plastic bags, nets, and a drum.[8] Unfortunately, the scary story doesn't stop there, as it isn't only animals that end up with plastic in their systems, but also we humans. First, due to the heat from the sun, microplastics leak out of the plastic items that float in the sea. These are eaten by plankton, which are eaten by small fish, which are eaten by crabs, oysters, and predatory fish, which are then eaten by humans, and, eventually, we inherit the toxic amount of microplastics into our body.

Plastic is also found in water bottles, and it's no wonder that 93 percent of adults have high levels of BPA in their urine. According to the Breast Cancer Fund Organisation, BPA has adverse health side effects, potentially causing birth defects, female infertility, increased risk for breast and prostate cancer, type 2 diabetes, and childhood obesity.

To ban plastic completely isn't a simple answer, because it's in nearly everything we do and buy. However, because I wish for our future generations to still experience the beautiful sea world, for our health to not be affected by mass plastic production, and for our children to understand the importance of plastic-free living, I've made a personal behaviour change and I invite you to do so as well. Here are my top to-do things to create a sustainable lifestyle benefiting my home, my health, and our environment.

- Use bamboo toothbrushes.
- Avoid menstrual pads and opt for period panties, widely available on the internet. Menstrual pads take five hundred years to degrade and are extremely harmful to the environment.
- Aim to purchase high-quality natural products, which mostly come in glass jars, rather than plastic, or at least in biodegradable plastic.
- Aim to purchase "green" household cleaning products, including liquid detergents, which mostly come in recyclable and biodegradable plastic bottles.
- Use recyclable and biodegradable garbage bags.
- Keep reusable grocery bags in your car at all times, or a couple of small reusable bags in your handbag if you walk around town.
- Buy your fruits and vegetables from farmers' markets and from grocery stores that allow you to fill your own jars with grains, nuts, and legumes.
- If it isn't possible to purchase from farmers' markets, reuse old plastic bags for weighing fruits and vegetables in the supermarket.
- Drink filtered water from the tap and avoid the use of plastic bottles. I drink Kangen water through my Enagic filter.
- Recycle your waste: glass, paper, plastic, and aluminium.
- Use recycled paper.
- Turn off all electrical sockets when not in use, to save energy and, of course, your electricity bill.
- Use ceramic pots for your plants.

You might already be doing some or all of the above. Either way, your awareness is heightened and you can always look for further ways to improve. I believe that your biggest achievement would be to encourage and motivate a friend, a family member, or even your children to also adopt one, a few, or all these ways to create a "greener" home. This ripple effect of positive action is the secret recipe for global change.

Transform the thought of *It doesn't matter what I do* into *I need to pay back to the environment that's hosting me right now*. We are all guests on planet Earth, and the way we've been behaving in the last one hundred years is changing the course of our planet's fate. I realised that instead of getting anxious about the consequences we will endure, instead of complaining about world politics and politicians' inability to provide global action, I prefer to focus on the love and hospitality that the planet provides. I want to be grateful for the blue sky, for the sun, for the moon, for the vast oceans and grand mountains, and the only way I can reciprocate this gratitude is by living a responsible, sustainable lifestyle. If I may, I would like to invite you to open up to this idea: Rather than be anxious about what the future holds, be grateful for the present natural beauty and live as if the planet's health is dependent upon you.

Reflections

For each of the home elements discussed earlier, rate how much needs to be done to improve it.

Home environment in general	Starting from zero	Still a lot to do	Small edits would be good	It's perfect!
Kitchen (ingredients you use)				
Bathroom (products you use)				
Household cleaning products				
Kitchen equipment				

Home environment in general	Starting from zero	Still a lot to do	Small edits would be good	It's perfect!
Nature at home (plants, feeding birds etc.)				
Home scent				
Radiation exposure				
Sustainability				

What is the one area or element of your home that requires most attention?

Which area or element of your home tends to decline after a period of progress? (E.g., a messy wardrobe, dying plants, inability to maintain sustainability)

What can you do to prevent falling into the old cycle again?

What's the one area or element in your home that energises you?

How can you enhance this area/element further, to get even more energy from it?

How will your physical and mental well-being be affected
if you improve all or some of the elements/areas of your
home?

Are you excited to try the Five-Week Home Awakening
Program? What excites you about it?

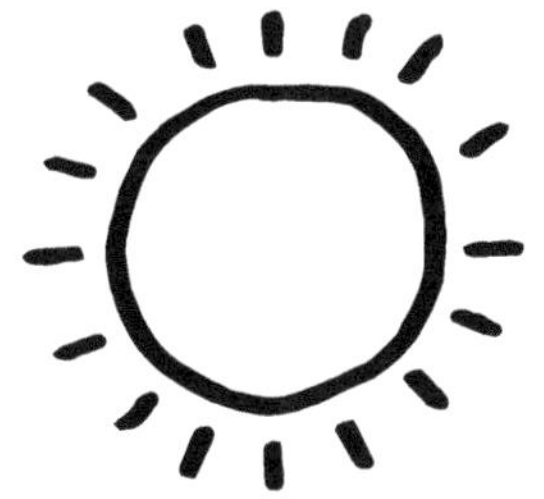

I prefer to focus
on the love
and hospitality
that the planet
provides.

Part 3

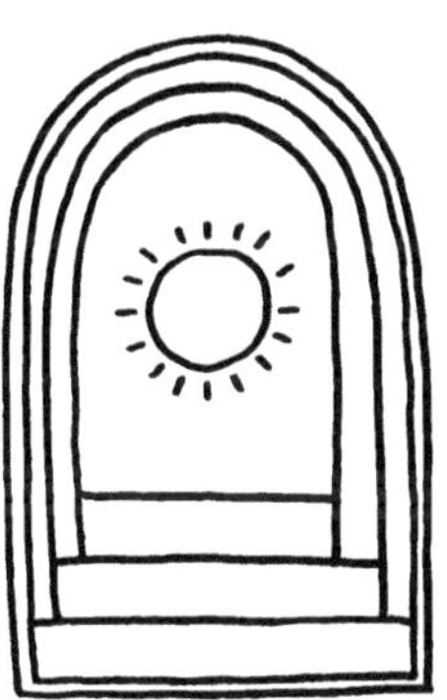

THE PROGRAM

WHAT IS THE PROGRAM?

It's a five-week program to cleanse, rearrange, and nourish every single corner of your home based on the knowledge you've gained from the previous sections of this book. During the program, we also focus on your nutrition and ME-time elements, which are far more easily carried out when the space you live in is inviting for these healthy activities. Throughout the program, you have the option to share the tasks with another house member, or you can do it all independently. Each week focuses on a specific room, and you will dedicate your thoughts and energy to that room only. As you move from space to space throughout the weeks, you will also have nutrition tasks and great recipes to support you. From week 3 onward, we introduce an element of ME time, when you start dedicating conscious time for your own self. It isn't as hard as it may seem; it is super fun, and remember, I'm always here with you.

WHAT IS THE GOAL OF THE PROGRAM?

As you might have understood, your general well-being depends not only on what you eat but also where you spend your recovery time. For most of us, home is where we are meant to rest, eat, sleep, and spend time with family. However, the home we live in might not provide us with the energy we require to live to our best potential. The goal of the program is just that: to create a home where you can repair, reenergise, be nourished, and pass this vital knowledge to the people around you and generations after you.

HOW SHOULD I APPROACH THE PROGRAM?

I suggest you read all the weeks upfront so you know what to expect and can dedicate some time to it. Once you start, answer the questions with a pencil and take it step by step. Remember, this program can be done over and over again; thus, some things that you've missed one time can be completed on your next approach. There's no pressure at all, so enjoy it and make sure to host a small social gathering at the end of the five weeks with your loved ones to celebrate your achievements!

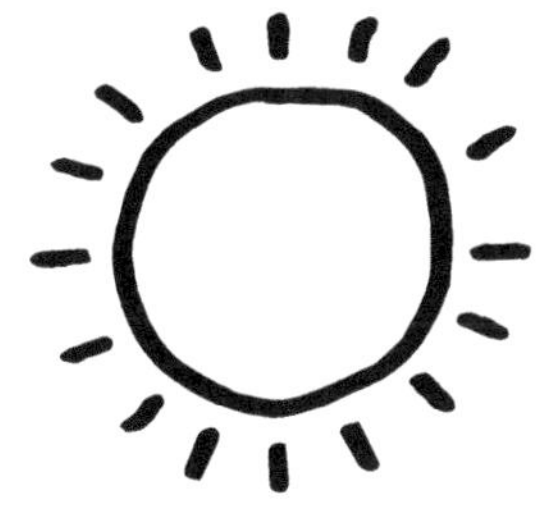

The goal is to create a home where you can repair, reenergise, be nourished, and pass this vital knowledge to the people around you.

Week One

The heart of the home—the kitchen

This first week focuses on helping you declutter your kitchen as well as helping you nourish it in a way that will support you in the coming weeks and complement your health. This is the reason we're targeting your kitchen first. The source of either health or disease, the kitchen is meant to be your temple where your body and mind feel safe to be nourished and rejuvenated with clean foods. In this first week, we will also focus on cleaning out your household cleaning products. Considering that this week is a kitchen detox, I also invite you to carry out a few simple detox recipes for your body. It would be fantastic if you coordinated week one from my book *Wake Up!* with this week, cleansing from within and out. However, following a few nutrition tips of the week from this book, along with other tasks, will be perfectly enough.

By the end of this week we should expect a healthy, "green", scented kitchen and a rejuvenated energised you!

8 steps to a clean "green"
healthy kitchen

STEP 1: STRUCTURED DECLUTTERING

Decluttering a space requires a bit of organisation and structure. I suggest dividing your kitchen into four parts, as simple as the figure below. Decide whether you want to go through all the parts, decluttering and rearranging in one day, or devote one day to one part.

Day:	Part 1	Part 3	Day:
Day:	Part 2	Part 4	Day:

STEP 2: GATHER ALL YOUR UNHEALTHY PRODUCTS

As you go through each part, remove the unhealthy ingredients listed on page 49. You'll feel ready to throw some products away and never buy them again, but with others, you may hesitate, and that's okay. Perhaps you just need a good healthy alternative for it to make that determined step.

I'm throwing away:

I'm still hesitant about:

STEP 3: ONE NEW PIECE OF KITCHEN EQUIPMENT?

If you still own a microwave, this is the time to take the plunge in disposing of the most convenient yet hazardous piece of kitchen equipment. Furthermore, decide if in the coming weeks, you would like to invest in just one item listed on page 76.

Microwave out?

New equipment in:

STEP 4: KITCHEN SCENT

Whether it's keeping a spray bottle with essential oils on the side or simmering spices, take the most desirable and convenient step for yourself in order to add a scent to your kitchen.

How do you plan to create a scent in the kitchen?

Introduce by which day?

STEP 5: PLANTS

Whether your kitchen is in direct or indirect sunlight or no light at all, there are always some plants that you can place around to freshen up the air, keep the place pretty, and make you smile.

Which plant/s?

Introduce by which day?

STEP 6: INTRODUCE SUSTAINABILITY

Aside from plastic, another key element to being a responsible guest on planet Earth is to save energy. Figure out which devices can be turned on only during use and off the rest of the time. In my kitchen, I control all my devices with one socket switch; therefore, I switch it on or off whenever I need to use something. My stove is also on only during use. Before I go to sleep, everything in the kitchen is off, except the fridge, of course. This first week is for you to get into that habit; perhaps sometimes you'll forget, but if you use this week to consciously implement this habit into your daily routine, soon you won't even need to think about it. Make sure to note your reduced electricity bill at the end of the month!

With regard to recycling, if you haven't started yet, this is the time to do it. You'll be amazed at the amount of packaging you can recycle. The next step will be to list where you reduce your use of plastic, whether it's investing in a reusable shopping bag or reusing old plastic bags; figuring out where can you buy legumes, grains, nuts, and powders package free; or finding local farmers' markets.

What's my current electricity bill?

Where can I cut down on plastic use?

STEP 7: "CLEAN" YOUR HOUSEHOLD CLEANING PRODUCTS

Because you read earlier about indoor pollution and how your household cleaning products could be the biggest contributor, in this first week of the program, you need to clear out all toxic products from your cupboards and replace them with either organic toxin-free products bought from the supermarket, or the simple alternatives listed on page 71. This includes liquid detergent for clothes washing.

I replace...	with...
Dishwasher detergent/ liquid	
Antibacterial solution (toilet seat & bowl)	
Glass / window cleaner	
Multi-surface floor cleaner	
Bathtub and shower cleaning paste	
Oven top / kitchen counter cleaner	
Washing machine detergent / liquid	

STEP 8: TIME FOR SHOPPING!

Time to set a day for shopping! It's no good throwing away unhealthy ingredients if you do not yet have an alternative. In fact, this is the reason so many people struggle to overcome old habits; there's no alternative to crowd them out. Here is an example shopping list of staple foods for your new healthy "green" kitchen.

Grains	Oils /Spices/ Condiments	Sweets /Dairy/Nuts/ Seeds
Brown rice / black rice	Coconut oil	Maple syrup
Quinoa	Olive oil	Raw honey
Buckwheat	Ghee butter	Coconut sugar
Amaranth		Stevia
Millet	Herbs & spices	Dairy
Rolled oats	Pink Himalayan salt	Kefir
Flours	Black pepper	Goat cheese
Oat flour	Cinnamon	Nut milk
Buckwheat flour	Turmeric	Nuts
Spelt flour	Whole cumin	Raw walnuts, cashews
Pasta	Star anise	Almonds, brazil nuts

Grains	Oils /Spices/ Condiments	Sweets /Dairy/Nuts/ Seeds
Wholegrain pasta	Cloves	Seeds
Quinoa pasta		Pumpkin seeds
Brown rice noodles	Other	Sunflower seeds
	Raw apple cider vinegar	Chia seeds / Flax seeds

Of course, it's important to buy all your products from trusted sources and preferably organic—not only fruits, vegetables, and meats, but also grains, spices, and other listed ingredients. Set a date in the first week for your shopping trip, and, if possible, find a place where you can purchase grains, legumes, nuts, and spices package free; instead, reuse your own bottles and jars. The above shopping list is just an example of how to structure your shopping list and gives you possible alternatives; however, you can always go back to page pages 29 and 49 and choose your own alternatives.

On this shopping day, you can also purchase the plant/s for the kitchen, the essential oils, and the "green" cleaning products.

What day am I going shopping?

STEP 1: MORNING APPLE CIDER VINEGAR (ACV)

Every morning, you can start with three to four glasses of water, and one glass can be mixed with 1 tablespoon of raw unfiltered ACV. Proven to have antibacterial properties, ACV also cleanses your skin, nourishes your digestive system, and boosts your immune system. Once opened, make sure to keep ACV in the fridge.

STEP 2: GREEN JUICE

Green juice recipes have incredible detox and cleansing properties. There are many recipes mixing vegetables with a fruit. However, to make things easy for you, I recommend that you have this green juice recipe every morning.

2 celery stalks
2 cucumbers
1 green apple
2 thin slices ginger

Better than your morning espresso, this juice will wake up all your cells and keep you at 100 percent for the rest of the day.

STEP 3: DETOX WATER

Drinking plenty of water is naturally detoxifying for the body, and I hope you're already drinking plenty of it! Introducing certain ingredients to water will add flavour and nourishing properties.

Try some of the suggestions given here and pick your favourite
to adopt into your daily routine. Putting the ingredients in a jar
of water allows you to refill the jar with more water throughout
the day. Please make sure to use organic ingredients, as it would
be a shame to have the right intention for drinking this water but
actually be drinking pesticides in liquid form.

Apple slices and cinnamon sticks
Lemon slices, handful of strawberries, and mint leaves
Orange wedges and a handful of blueberries
Orange wedges and raspberries
Ginger slices and fresh or frozen mango

Week One Reflections

I sincerely hope you enjoyed the start of the program and are happy with the results! Before we get on with week two, take some time to reflect and write down your experiences. A week ago, you might have been feeling completely different than you do today, and it's important to note these changes in order to feel progress and be motivated to continue.

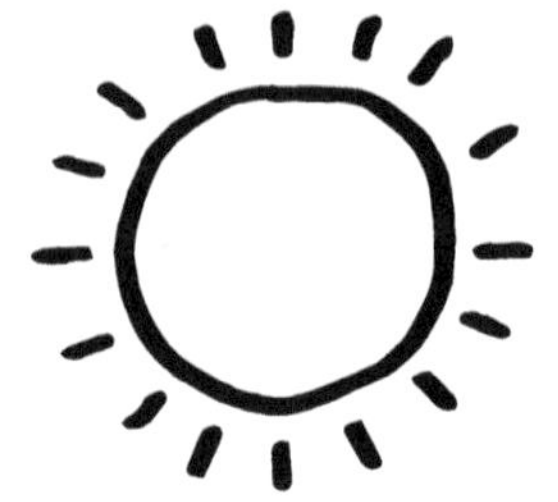

The kitchen is
meant to be
your temple where
your body and
mind feel safe to
be nourished and
rejuvenated with
clean foods.

Week Two

The soul of the home—the bedroom

My bedroom is my most favourite part of the house. It's a place to rest, relax, and feel safe from the outside world. In the same way as we did in week one, we'll now target the bedroom by decluttering and nourishing it with positive energy through plants, scents, and reducing radiation exposure. Through the guided steps on how and what to do, at the end of the week, you'll sense the different vibe in your bedroom. The moment you walk into it, you'll feel very calm, your sleep will become deep and uninterrupted, and your mornings will be fresher and happier!

8 steps to a "Zen" bedroom

STEP 1: STRUCTURED DECLUTTERING

Divide your room into four parts and decide when each part will be decluttered and organised. It may take you a day or more but, most importantly, don't jump from one part to another. Make sure to complete one part before starting another.

Day:	Part 1	Part 3	Day:
Day:	Part 2	Part 4	Day:

STEP 2: THE PROCESS OF DECLUTTERING

Clothes, more clothes, and even more clothes. It's a very human habit to always want more. I used to be that person who said, "I have nothing to wear!" although my wardrobe was bursting with clothes. Sound familiar? Did you also notice how we tend to wear the same thing all the time, even though the options in our wardrobe are endless? One of the reasons is because we simply can't see the rest of our clothes due to the mess in the wardrobe! Take out all your clothes, throw them on the bed, and decide, item by item, whether you'll wear it or not, whether you still like it or not, or whether it's even still your style. Styles change over time, and something that you wore a few years ago perhaps no longer suits you or doesn't make you happy anymore. Be very honest with yourself when considering each piece of clothing and wonder if someone else would benefit from it more than you. Some clothes you'll be hesitant about; for these, I suggest laying them on a chair or some other very obvious place. If you don't wear them in the next seven days, you'll never wear them.

When I divide my bedroom into four parts, I look at each
item in every part and ask myself: "Does it make me smile? Or
does it cause no emotion? Or does it actually bring up negative
associations/memories?" Of course, anything that causes negative
associations should be thrown out or given away immediately, as it's
hindering the positive energy in the room. If it causes no emotion,
I also tend to get rid of it, but it is up to you to decide whether
you need that item or not. Remember, your bedroom is a place
of rest and love, not a place for collecting items that gather dust
and pollute your air. I'm very brutal when it comes to bedroom
decluttering and do this process every six months, as that's enough
time for some clutter to pile up. Looking through each part of the
room, write down the items and their associated emotions.

What items in the bedroom make you happy?

What items in the bedroom make you sad?

STEP 3: THE PROCESS OF ARRANGING

Once you've collected bags (hopefully many!) for charity, recycling, and general waste, you now have the chance to arrange everything that's left in a way that will create even more space. My best suggestion is to read the book *The Life-Changing Magic of Tidying Up* by Marie Kondo, who teaches you her Japanese way of decluttering, arranging things, folding clothes, and much more. The secret I learned is to have all your clothes in the wardrobe be visible. Since I've adopted this method, I feel no need for more shopping; I have more than enough.

STEP 4: PLANTS

As you remove unnecessary items from the room and get rid of clothes that are never worn, you create more space for positive vibes to enter. And let these vibes come from green plants that will clean up the air, absorb any toxicity, and fill every corner of the room with love and energy. Placed next to your bed, by the window, and in all other corners of the room, they'll make sure to keep you safe, as long as you provide them with the love they need.

Which plant/s?

Introduce by which day?

STEP 5: BEDROOM SCENT

This should be a gentle scent to remind you of the "zen" mood of the room. I like to use a spray bottle with a mix of gentle essential oils, right before I go to sleep, so the scent follows me into my dreams. I love how these small details, no matter the mood, make us smile and awaken all our senses. Choose your way. Refer to page 81 to pick your way to add a scent to your home, and implement it this week. Remember, if you do use candles, choose the right quality, and it's best to put them out before you go to sleep.

How do you plan to create a scent in the bedroom?

STEP 6: RADIATION EXPOSURE

Now it's time to target your attachment to your phone, tablet, and/or TV in the bedroom. Count how many devices that emit electromagnetic fields are currently in your bedroom. If none, you're the hero and can already help someone else who sleeps with their TV on, with their phone next to their head, and so on. Read the section again on radiation exposure and its dangers for the body (page 83). I believe the information is rather convincing to encourage you or someone else to act. I have a no-device policy for our bedroom: no laptops, no phones, no TV. I put my mobile phone on airplane mode, leave it in the living room, and retire to my "sanctuary"—my bedroom. I cuddle with my partner or my dogs (depending on who is available!) or read a book before falling asleep.

The addiction of scrolling down our phone before sleep has detached us from reality, from real sensations, and feelings. Furthermore, as soon as we open our eyes, we pick up the radiated device into our fragile hands just awakened from sleep, force our eyes to read the news or messages, and force our just-awakened brain to process the information. What effect do you think that has on your physical and mental well-being? So, this week's task is to help you come back to your senses and cleanse your room from any possible radiation. Once you successfully complete this task in this week, you'll be able to see the difference in your sleep and good mood in the mornings, which will encourage you to continue with it.

What devices do you currently have or have the habit of bringing into the room?

How do you plan to reduce or completely eliminate radiation exposure when you're in the bedroom?

What day this week will this plan be activated fully?

STEP 7: SUSTAINABILITY

Simple tasks such as having the light off when not in the room, or switching off the sockets when not in use, can save electricity. It may sound rather simple yet can be dismissed, especially by younger generations. Take time to perfect this yourself, and teach the younger ones about the importance of saving electricity.

You can continue the nutrition advice from week 1 and try the following steps for a nourishing, strong week.

STEP 1: BREAKFAST OF A CHAMPION

Even though it's a very important meal, breakfast tends to be skipped. The excuse is always "no time" or "not hungry". The people who say this are also the people who struggle to lose weight, feel tired during the day, and tend to be heavy coffee drinkers. Imagine: Your body hasn't eaten since dinner, which is at least eight or nine hours ago, then you skip breakfast. This will leave your body without any nourishment for another three or four hours, except for coffee. This could be viewed as intermittent fasting, but there's a few problems with that. One is that it cannot be done every day, driving your body to extreme hunger and frequent headaches. Eventually, when you do eat, the meal is too large and shoots your insulin excessively high. You start eating more in the afternoon and evening as your body requires the energy to function, which disrupts your sleep and delays your wake-up time. So, yet again, you rush to work without eating any breakfast, and the vicious cycle goes on and on.

I hope that this week of daily conscious breakfast preparation will eventually lead to mornings where you jump out of bed because you so look forward to eating your delicious breakfast. I invite you to follow the breakfast plan for the week, and it would be even more fun if other members of the house joined you in the challenge.

Day 1	Chia Seed Pudding (page 171)
Day 2	Omelette with Veggies (page 172)
Day 3	Oat Porridge (page 172)
Day 4	Egg Wrap (page 173)
Day 5	Breakfast Bowl (page 174)
Day 6	Homemade Granola (page 175)
Day 7	Acai Bowl (page 175)

If you're preparing breakfast with someone else, whether it's your partner or a child, there are always tasks you can delegate. And if you're still drinking the green juice from week one, and you add one of these delicious breakfasts, you'll set yourself up for a very energetic successful day. Trust me on that!

STEP 2: HEALTHY SNACKS

Snacking is the reason for many of our troubles, if you do it wrong. As I'm writing this book, I'm snacking! It's a habit of a writer, I guess, but even more so for people always sitting at their desks. Working eight or nine hours a day can be so tiring and limiting in action that the least a person can do is have some flavourful entertainment in their mouth. Of course, drinking water (especially the flavoured water from week one) can distract bored senses for a while, yet a good alternative to snacking can never be too much.

Try the snack recipes from the Recipe section (page 187) for this week and be sure to share!

Week Two Reflections

This is possibly my favourite week because I just love a clean, unclogged, relaxed bedroom. This is where the magic is supposed to happen, and I sincerely hope that you now feel it too. Perhaps it might take you longer than this one week and that's absolutely fine. Go at your own pace and enjoy this period of cleansing and nourishing every corner of your home. Share your experiences and feelings with yourself here. Every time you do this program (as mentioned earlier, you could do it every six months or more often), the experience will be more familiar and even more profound.

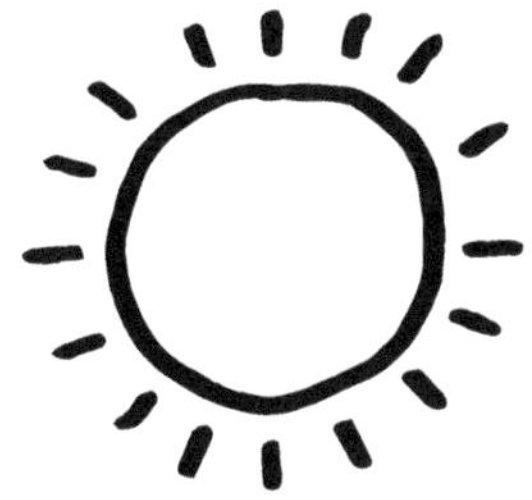

I love how these small details, no matter the mood, make us smile and awaken all our senses.

Week Three

The centre of your home—the living room

The living room is a place where we spend most of our time—watching TV, lazing around on the couch, greeting our guests, eating family dinners, and so on. If you look around your living room now, what energy does it hold? Dull or vibrant? Calm or hectic? Clean or messy? It's up to you what energy you want to fill your space with, something that makes you smile and want to have people over at your place to share the beautiful atmosphere you've created. My living room space is rather calm, clean, and harmonious. I wouldn't call it vibrant or flamboyant, yet it's lively in its own peaceful way. It's very similar to my own character and personal energy, and that's why when I come home, I truly feel that I'm home.

Perhaps this week, you'll still be completing some tasks from the previous weeks, or maybe you're already sitting in your living room wondering about the first step of week three? Very similar to previous weeks, first we divide the living room into four parts and start to declutter, cleanse, and nourish every part at your own pace.

7 steps to a spacious living room

STEP 1: STRUCTURED DECLUTTERING

Divide your living room into four parts, and assign the time and date for each part:

Day:	Part 1	Part 3	Day:
Day:	Part 2	Part 4	Day:

STEP 2: THE PROCESS OF DECLUTTERING

By now, you should be a master of decluttering! Remember, whatever doesn't make you smile needs to be removed from your home. Each part of the living room deserves your full attention; take your time and avoid rushing through it. You may have a shelf of unorganised paperwork, bills, and admin things. Make yourself a nice cup of tea and go through it all, either recycling unnecessary papers or creating files and organising each paper for its purpose. A stack of paperwork carries a very unpleasant energy: neglected, forgotten, not accepted. And that energy will represent itself in your body in the form of a tight knot. The moment your papers are organised, you'll feel lighter and a sense of freedom will come over your body. I find it so fascinating how the simple act of decluttering can have such an immense impact on how we feel. Similar to week two, I would like you to look at each item and experience the feeling it gives you. Depending on how it makes you feel, decide to either eliminate it from your space or keep it.

What items in the living room make you happy?

What items in the living room make you sad?

What items in the living room cause no emotion?

STEP 3: THE PROCESS OF ARRANGING

Allow your creative fluids to overflow and arrange your things the way you want. I believe that because I went to a boarding school, I grew to love having posts/photos on my wall: old photos of family members, postcards from the cities I visited, small mementoes, basically anything that makes me smile, and if I can stick it on the wall, even better. I like to use Blu Tack, because it doesn't ruin the wall paint or paper.

Arranging each part of the room should take into consideration dust collection, ease of cleaning, a tidy decluttered look, and, of course, your emotions. I support the minimalist style; the fewer dust-collecting items you have, the better. However, it can be difficult to throw away souvenirs that hold memories, and that's why I prefer to stick things on the wall! Dedicating an area or a shelf for souvenirs is also a great idea to gather the positive energy in one place; it also makes it easier to clean, especially if it's an enclosed glass cabinet. It's really up to you how you arrange your items and shelves, but one thing this program requires you to do is to be conscious in your arrangements and not place things just for the sake of it. Every item in your home has a meaning and has its own place. I invite you to enliven your living room with your best creativity. This is also a perfect week to get other house members involved and enjoy some bonding time, whether it's your partner or child. Children love to help and be asked for their opinion, only we do it so rarely that we tend to dismiss their early wisdom.

STEP 4: PLANTS

According to some studies, we should have two plants for every 100 square feet of an area. Get your calculator out and count how many plants you require in order to really freshen up the air in the room. One plant won't do the job! Get ready to create a jungle in your living room and you'll notice the improvement of allergies, headaches, and even mood. You can go back to page 79 and pick which specific plants you want, and, of course, you're free to choose your own. Remember, the leafier they are, the better!

Which plant/s?

Introduce by which day?

STEP 5: LIVING ROOM SCENT

Have you already decided which scent you want to represent your home? The living room is where guests gather, and you want them to feel a tingle of emotions: a sense of calm and comfort, a sense of familiarity and trust. It will be difficult for your friends to leave your home after experiencing all these inviting elements of your new healthy home! There's no pressure to always have some sort of smell in the living room; perhaps you can do it when you are expecting visitors or when you're spending some time in the living room. A simple way is to burn incense, which will reach every corner of the room. However, some incense can cause headaches, therefore, it's important to try various types. My suggestion is to start with the lightest one. My favourite incense scent is a mix of berries and greens. Remember to invest in high quality incense and play around with the smells this week.

How do you plan to create a scent in the living room?

Introduce by which day?

STEP 6: RADIATION EXPOSURE

Which devices do you have in your living room? TV, Wi-Fi router, computer, wireless printer, and so on. All, of course, are emitting electromagnetic fields, and by now we already know the severity of the problem. This week, let's try to decrease the radiation exposure as much as possible. For example, turn on your TV at the socket only when you're watching it; otherwise, have it switched off. Turn off your Wi-Fi router before going to bed, power off your laptop, or, instead of having wireless internet, switch to a hardwired internet connection. For more examples, you can read through the section on page 83 again.

What devices do you currently have and have the habit of always keeping on in the living room?

How do you plan to reduce or completely eliminate radiation exposure in the living room?

What day this week will this plan be activated fully?

STEP 7: SUSTAINABILITY

Putting the plug into the sockets of electric devices only when you need them is a great way to save electricity—and lower your bill! Some homes have a switch to turn the socket on or off, so all you have to do is to switch it off whenever you aren't using something. I must admit it isn't easy to remember this, and you might also struggle to keep other house members in check; however, persistence is a virtue! It's just a matter of conscious effort and practice. After all, there's a bigger reason why we're doing all of this.

Decrease your purchase of cheap plastic products and even souvenirs and try to support small enterprises that have handmade meaningful products. Always recycle your paper and buy notepads and even printing paper made of recycled paper.

Trying to introduce conscious sustainability into every aspect of your life will create a very pleasant relationship between you and Mother Earth: a reciprocal respect.

INTRODUCING ME TIME

ME time means time away from outside noise and fostering a deep connection with your inner world. Sometimes, we're so stuck in the routine, looking after everyone else, that we forget our own needs and desires; we forget how we like to relax and even how we like to spend time. I have to admit that I get lost in translation too, working hard, looking after my clients, spending time with family, and lots of social time with friends. Even though I find it all enjoyable, I'm giving away quite a lot of energy, and, after some time, I feel somewhat depleted. That's why it's important to dedicate a minimum of two to three hours a week for ME time, when you contain your energy within and allow your body to focus on recharging. ME time can encompass so many types of activity; it's really up to you. However, the requirement is that you're alone in an activity that doesn't require too much energy (e.g., reading, writing, meditation, knitting, painting, massages, foot self-reflexology, and light yoga or breathing exercises). The task for the week is that you find one hour on three days this week to dedicate to yourself. If you're really tight on time, perhaps it could be thirty minutes in the morning and thirty minutes in the evening. Whatever it takes, I invite you to make a conscious effort to choose an activity and dedicate a time to recharge.

How much ME time do you usually get?

Which **ME**-time activities would you like to introduce this week? Choose activities that recharge you and make you feel good.

Give yourself a detailed plan on how you'll spend your three hours of ME time this week. Day? Time? Activity?

First 1 hour	Second 1 hour	Third 1 hour
What day?	What day?	What day?
What time?	What time?	What time?

First 1 hour	Second 1 hour	Third 1 hour
What?	What?	What?

Nutrition advice for the week

Keeping up your favourite tasks from the two previous weeks, now we'll introduce two new elements this week: baking and dinner. I understand that you may be feeling overwhelmed with all these tasks in one week, so take your time. This program is here to guide you and not pressure you. I'm with you all the way, and I hope you can feel it!

HEALTHY BAKING

In the Recipe section, you'll find a selection of baking recipes. Each recipe gives a sequence of steps, some of which you can delegate to a child or friend. Nothing better than to chat, bake, and eat the result with a cup of herbal tea! Who said that baked items must come with a load of sugar, milk, and wheat? After I have encouraged you to "healthy bake", you may go even further by following other "healthy bake" recipes, or even create your own.

DINNER TIME

What do you usually eat for dinner? I know two extremes: skipping the meal or eating a lot at dinner because that is the only big meal of the day. Neither of the extremes serves your body well. I propose having a selection of recipes that can be prepared for each evening, and any leftovers can be eaten the next day. Cooking dinner can be quite a lot, especially if you've just come back from work or have had a long busy day, so it's tempting to order a takeaway or end up eating bread, cheese, and yoghurt. But I promise you, it doesn't have to be complicated. Try out my recipes and decide for yourself!

Suggested dinner plan for the week (you have the freedom to swap the recipes around).

Day 1	Eggplant and Chickpea Hot Pot (page 179)
Day 2	Seabass Pineapple Coconut Curry (page 180)
Day 3	Baked Sweet Potato with Vegetable Stuffing (page 181)
Day 4	Baked Vegetables with Brown Rice (page 182)
Day 5	Lentil and Sweet Potato Hot Pot (page 183)
Day 6	Beetroot Burgers with Lettuce Wraps (page 184)
Day 7	Roasted Cauliflower with Buckwheat and Avocado Slices (page 185)

Week Three Reflections

This must be your favourite activity. Share your experiences and your challenges to reach the goal of a new spacious living room. Let yourself know where you exceeded your expectations and where you required more time and improvement. How are the other house members, if any, reacting to your participation in the program? Write, write, write.

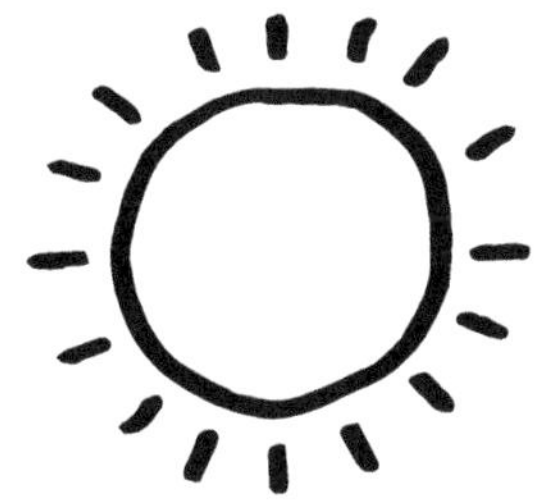

Dull or vibrant?
Calm or hectic?
Clean or messy?
It's up to you
what energy you
want to fill your
space with.

Week Four

Where the job gets done—the bathroom

The bathroom is no different to any other room. It also requires decluttering and nourishing simply because, in the bathroom, you cleanse and nourish your skin, the largest organ in the body. We've talked about the danger of commercial products and which natural alternatives you can use, so I believe you now have an idea what this week is all about.

A very interesting observation that a friend once made is the misconception that once you lead a healthy lifestyle, your bills shoot up. I've noticed the complete opposite, especially in the area of beauty and cosmetics. How much money do you spend on self-care and beauty? Now consider the following: Are those products and treatments natural and chemical free? I personally don't purchase perfume, paint my nails, dye my hair, purchase any makeup, or have a hundred different plastic bottles for skin care. It's also easy when I travel because I only have one soap for my face, one soap for my hair, face oil, and a natural SPF cream. It is scary to think how much money I've spent on beauty products and treatments previously, but now I know best what my skin needs. Shall we go ahead and start the work?

STEP 1: STRUCTURED DECLUTTERING

Divide the bathroom into 4 parts. If you have more than one bathroom, the process is the same for all!

Day:	Part 1	Part 3	Day:
Day:	Part 2	Part 4	Day:

STEP 2: PROCESS OF DECLUTTERING

Any bottle whose ingredients contain words you can't pronounce should really be eliminated from your space and away from your skin. Go back to the basics. Think, would your great-grandmother use this? Will your organs be happy with ingesting benzene and various other chemicals? Collect all the "bad" products (see page 62) on one side and natural on the other. If you're confused whether an item is natural or not, research the ingredients on the internet and make your final call on it. Some unhealthy items you won't be able to part with, and that's okay; just know that there's a natural alternative to absolutely everything.

What items in the bathroom are natural?

What items in the bathroom are unnatural?

STEP 3: PROCESS OF ARRANGING

I could imagine that after step 2, your bathroom might be looking pretty empty. Not to worry; it's time to get those alternatives from page 66. I understand it can be rather difficult to switch from one thing to another in such a short time; therefore, take your time. Try new chemical-free products, try natural soaps, and, eventually, you'll find exactly what your body needs. What I dream of is for everyone to realise that whatever they put on their body, on their nails, in their hair, absolutely matters. Of course, we want to be beautiful, but does that have to come at such a high cost?

Share here how you have found alternatives for your usual daily self-care products:

Unhealthy, full of chemicals	Healthy, natural alternative

STEP 4: BATHROOM SCENT

You're already at a stage, I hope, that you don't use air fresheners, toilet fresheners, etc. If you have a window in your bathroom, then that's the best way to freshen the air. However, for most of us, the bathroom can be quite damp and not carry a pleasant smell, especially after a toilet visit. One of the oldest tricks to get rid of any smell in the bathroom is to burn a single match—works like magic! If your bathroom collects too much dampness, the easiest way to control it is to put a dehumidifier for an hour or so in the bathroom after you've showered, which will control the level of moisture in the air.

To introduce a scent to a bathroom, you can choose from incense to naturally scented candles or keep a spray bottle with essential oils. You have the freedom to create, so go ahead!

How do you plan to create a scent in the bathroom?

Introduce by which day?

STEP 5: SUSTAINABILITY

How about recycled toilet paper? Of course, it isn't made out of already used toilet paper but, instead, from postconsumer recycled content such as receipts, tags, labels, and paper. It's a great way to save the trees, save energy, and keep the water clean; however, it has been found that recycled toilet paper has small traces of BPA (which originally come from credit card receipts). This is too little to be worried about, and recycled toilet paper is a much better option than purchasing new toilet paper.

Instead of buying a plastic toothbrush, which will sit in a landfill forever after you've used it, convert to a bamboo toothbrush that is biodegradable and will decompose into the soil in no time once you have thrown it away. Not only is it healthier for the environment but it also contains bristles that can get rid of bacteria and stains from your teeth on a microscopic level. The recommended lifespan of a bamboo toothbrush is also around three months, after which you can compost it yourself or throw it into a composting commercial bin. Easy purchase, if you ask me!

And, of course, there are the numerous plastic bottles/containers for gels, shampoos, creams, oils, and so on. Sometimes it's very difficult to find products that come in a glass jar; however, some natural beauty companies make a conscious effort to not only nourish your skin but also keep the planet happy. I use bar soaps for my body and hair; therefore, I avoid plastic bottles. Whatever little bit you can do counts!

How do you plan to increase the sustainability of your bathroom?

Nutrition advice for skin and hair

Unlike other weeks when we had to focus on nourishing ourselves from within, now we'll focus on nourishing the skin and hair from the outside, which is equally as important. I remember as a ten-year-old kid with beautiful long brown hair, my mom used to nourish my hair with natural products she prepared in the kitchen. I continue this habit today and remember converting many girls at school and university to my mother's old beauty ways.

No matter if you are male or female, everybody needs to pay a little attention to their skin. I'll talk more about skin health and how we can avoid skin ageing in my next book, but until then, try to introduce these few steps to feel the difference and keep you wanting more.

HAIR CARE: MAMA'S ORIGINAL HAIR TREATMENT

For my female readers, you can't go wrong with this recipe. If you do it regularly once a week, you will notice hair growth, volume, shine, softness, and an overall healthy look. I have been doing this hair treatment for over fifteen years and absolutely love it. Doesn't matter what type of hair you have or whether your scalp is dry or oily, this recipe is good for all.

2 egg yolks
1 to 2 tablespoons honey
1 teaspoon olive oil
Few drops lemon juice

Mix the ingredients in a bowl, apply to your hair, massage it into the roots and all along the hair, cover with a shower cap then an old head scarf, and leave it in for 45 minutes to 2 hours. Wash off with water and your natural shampoo or soap. Repeat once a week. There are many variations to this recipe, but this is the foundation of them all. Get familiar with it, do it regularly, and, by the time you'll want more, you can get my book on skin and hair beauty. It's also a great way to have bonding time for mothers with their daughters or a fun girlfriend time.

BODY CARE: MOISTURISER FROM THE KITCHEN

If you're a body type that gets hot very easily, then I recommend smothering cold-pressed coconut oil all over your body after you've had a shower. Conversely, if you're a body type that gets cold very easily, then cold-pressed sesame oil will invigorate your blood circulation and keep you warm. I tend to use sesame oil more, but on hot summer days, I switch to coconut oil. Moisturising yourself with these oils may sound strange, but trust me, it only takes around 5 minutes for the body to absorb the oils and your skin will be left smooth and nourished. And this is the week for you to try it out.

FACIAL CARE: FACE MASK TO SUIT EACH TYPE

One of my mom's favourite facial care routines is to first exfoliate with an oatmeal mask and then apply a gentle moisturising chocolate face mask. Yes, you read it right! Chocolate face mask… try not to be around people who are chocolate lovers!

Oat mask	Chocolate mask
1 tablespoon milled oats	1 tablespoon melted dark chocolate
1 tablespoon olive oil	1 tablespoon honey
1 egg white	1 tablespoon your own thick facial cream
Few drops lemon juice	

Mix the ingredients of each mask in separate bowls. First apply the oat mask. Leave it on for 20 minutes until dry and then wash it off with warm water. Afterward, apply the chocolate mask, leave it on for 20 to 30 minutes and then wash it off with warm water. Repeat this routine once a week. Before you apply either of the masks, put on a little bit on your face to check if you have any allergic reaction to it.

Whether you're female or male, your skin is unisex and has equal requirements for treatment and care. In week four, these treatments can be done in your dedicated ME time hours!

When do you plan to carry out the above self-care treatments?

Week Four Reflections

We're nearing the end of the journey! This week was a lot about the products you apply on your skin, hair, and teeth. Share the experiences of this week, challenges, and improvements, and what has actually been your favourite thing so far out of all four weeks?

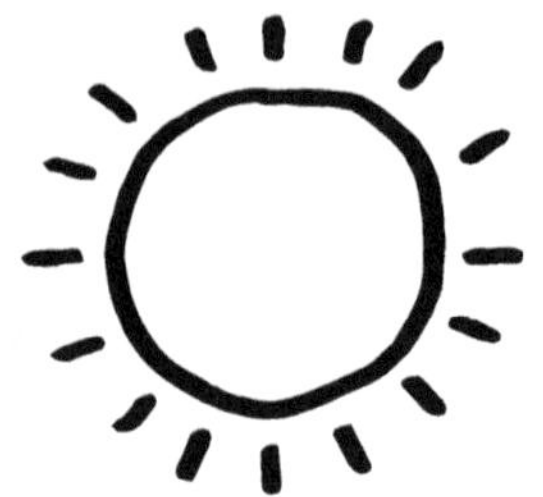

Whatever
little bit
you can do
counts!

Week Five

Settle in your beautiful new space

In this last week of the program, I leave some space for you to organise any other room in your house in the exact same manner as you did the previous rooms. It could be your office, a guest room, storage, or a child's room. My suggestion is to tackle your child's room together with your child: Get them involved in dividing the room into four parts, dedicating a day and time to each part, and going through each part, asking questions such as: Does this item make me happy? Can someone else benefit from this item? Give your child the opportunity to choose their own scent and plant for the room with the condition that this plant is now the child's responsibility. It's a really fun and engaging process for child and adult alike.

This final week is also for you to set in stone all the learned habits, such as watering plants, infusing scents into the room, recycling, switching off the plugs, reducing radiation exposure, and, of course, cooking with all your new healthy ingredients. By now, it should all come very naturally to you.

INTRODUCING MEDITATION

Considering that your home by now carries a completely different energy than it had four weeks ago, I propose that you now focus on enhancing your ME time by introducing two to three minutes of meditation rituals. If you are already meditating daily, then after this program your meditation experience will be even more profound with all the decluttered space and natural smells. If you haven't quite mastered it yet, then now is the time to try.

Find a corner in the house where you feel most relaxed, sit on a cushion, keep your spine straight, close your eyes, and start with long deep belly breathing. Set a timer to 15 seconds, and with time you can increase this time to 30 seconds, 1 minute, 3 minutes, and so on. If your mind wanders, bring it back to your breath.

My personal routine regarding meditation is connected to kundalini yoga taught by Yogi Bhajan. I choose a meditation that feels right to me for the page that I am on and practice it for forty days consecutively. It takes forty days to change a habit. If you are open to exploring different ways, then search the internet and YouTube for kundalini yoga classes and meditations. I highly recommend Guru Jagat, Gurmukh, and the 3HO YouTube channel. In my first book, *Wake Up!*, I provide different kundalini exercises and meditations for every week of the programme; if you still don't have my first book then it's time to grab your copy.

Where and how would you like to carry out your meditation routine?

I also propose that you dedicate thirty minutes on another two days of the week for brisk walking. Nothing beats the benefits of fast walking. Make sure your head is looking forward not down, your shoulders are pushing back, and your chest is forward. Walk with confidence and aim. That way, you have physical activity four days of the week, which is the perfect healthy balance.

How do you plan to introduce and maintain your physical activity? With which exercises?

INTRODUCING EXERCISE

Sometimes, people have the misconception that they have to exercise every day to see results. Of course, daily exercise is good, but the problem is that your body gets tired and you get bored. Therefore, I always recommend exercising two to three times a week; that way, it can be sustainable over months. I'm not a big advocate of gyms; I believe you can do a lot at home alone or with a buddy. From what I've experienced from analysing my clients' physical bodies is that gym equipment stiffens the body and tends to mainly focus on large muscle groups. Many people are reluctant to attend the gym or group classes because they think they're weak, not flexible, or not athletic enough. Well, we have to start somewhere, right?

All you need is thirty to forty minutes on two days of the week, a yoga mat, resistance and elastic bands, and you're set for success. You can access some great free YouTube videos with workouts, and once you feel a need for more, start attending group classes with more confidence and strength. Sharing those thirty to forty minutes of exercise with a partner, friend, or your child is best!

Week Five Reflections

Here we are! You have completed the final week of the program. Share your thoughts about this week and its own challenges with regards to sticking to a meditation and exercise routine. And of course, once you're done, remember to celebrate your achievements, and what better way to celebrate than share the joy with your close friends and loved ones?

Remember to celebrate your achievements, and what better way to celebrate than share the joy with your close friends and loved ones?

For all the home elements improved throughout the program, rate each one according to how you feel about it now. Compare your answers to the answers you gave on page 91.

Home environment in general	Very dull, messy	Could be better	Small edits would be good	It's perfect!
Kitchen (ingredients you use)				
Bedroom				
Living room				
Bathroom (products you use)				
Household cleaning products				
Kitchen equipment				
Nature at home (plants, feeding birds, etc.)				

Home environment in general	Very dull, messy	Could be better	Small edits would be good	It's perfect!
Home scent				
Radiation exposure				
Sustainability				

What is now your favourite space in your home?

Which part of your home requires more work and energy?

When do you plan to go through the program again?

How has this program affected your general well-being?

How do you plan to encourage others to live a sustainable life for the well-being of our planet?

How has the program affected your relationship with
other people?

How do you plan to maintain the new energy in your home?

What to Do After the Program

The sole intention of this book and program is to show you the extensive impact a home environment can have on your mental and physical health, and on the people around you. Remember that you're creating a safe home environment not just for yourself but also for future generations and for the health of our planet. It is time to start living a conscious lifestyle that is respectful of the future and grateful for the present.

You can repeat the five-week program or just one of the weeks every five to six months or even more often. It is always good to cleanse, nourish, re-energise, and every time you do it you will have an even deeper experience. At times, when you feel out of balance, down, or anxious, take time to carry out one or all of the weeks. It will help you clear your mind and see things from a new perspective.

When your kitchen is healthy and you have set rules about what healthy ingredients and foods you can buy, you have the flexibility to have cheat meals outside of your home. I talk about the 80/20 rule in my previous book, *Wake Up!*, in which 80 percent of the time you are healthy with a 20 percent window for cheat meals. We can apply this recommendation to our new healthy home style: whenever I'm at home, I eat healthy; whenever I'm out, I have the flexibility to nourish myself differently if I choose.

After reading this book, I hope you have realised that it is not all about food and nutrition. Paying attention to your mobile phone attachment and your exposure to radiation is vital for your overall well-being. What about eliminating as much plastic as possible from your life? What about the level of indoor pollution in your home? Many more questions should now arise within your mind, and the more you ask, the more meticulous you will become about everything you purchase. The more aware you become, the more conscious your life will become.

This book has provided you with a complete guide on how to protect yourself in every aspect of life, and I sincerely wish for you to pass this knowledge on to your close friends and loved ones.

As a nutrition and lifestyle expert, I believe one can achieve an equilibrium in life by leading a conscious lifestyle. It is natural and absolutely normal to fall in and out of equilibrium; however, it is important to know when and how you can find your way back to balance—and this cannot be achieved anywhere better than within the walls of your own home, within the palace of your own creation.

Until the next book,
Nigora

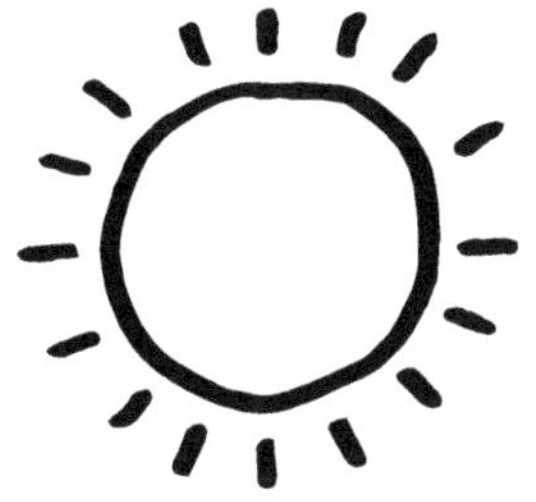

I believe
one can achieve
an equilibrium
in life by leading
a conscious
lifestyle.

Recipe section

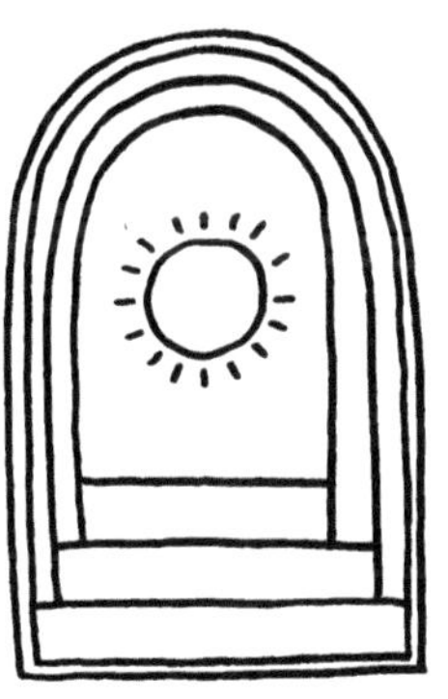

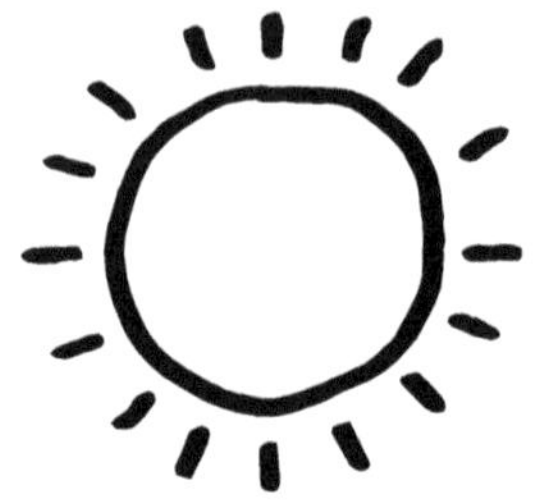

The more aware
you become,
the more conscious
your life
will become.

You may be familiar with my cooking style and have already tried the recipes in *Wake Up!* In this book, you'll find a broader choice of vegetarian options, a little more flavour, and a little more creativity. Some of the recipes I've taken from my time at the Rouxbe Culinary School, and some come from my all-time favourite recipe app, "Green Kitchen", which I highly recommend! I strongly recommend you use organic items most of the time; the flavour of your food will be so much more enhanced.

As a side note, I would love to see how you prepare these recipes and the results you achieve with your cooking, so post the photos of your meals on Instagram with the hashtag #nigorarecipes and I will definitely comment and motivate you further!

Breakfast

This is the best meal of the day, so put effort into it. At first, it may seem too difficult to follow the recipes and the last thing you want to do early in the morning. However, you can perhaps practice on the weekends, prep the ingredients the night before, or simply wake up a little early (chuckle)! The point is that, after some time, you'll become a master and will start creating your own amazing recipes.

Chia Pudding – (kid-friendly recipe)

Ingredients
50–70 grams blueberries, raspberries, or any other berry
3 tablespoons chia seeds
250 ml almond milk
1 teaspoon freshly ground cardamom
Pinch sea salt
Toppings: 4 tablespoons Greek-style yoghurt, sliced banana,
1 tablespoon maple syrup, sunflower seeds, sesame seeds,
walnuts

Directions
Mash the berries with a fork and mix with the chia seeds, almond milk, cardamom, and salt. Let it sit for about 20 minutes, then place in a serving bowl and add the yoghurt. In a separate bowl, mix the banana slices with the maple syrup, seeds, and walnuts. Add this mixture to the chia yoghurt bowl. Mix well and enjoy.

Omelette with Veggies

Ingredients

Olive or coconut oil

½ onion, diced

1 garlic clove, minced

3 or 4 cherry tomatoes, diced

3 or 4 button mushrooms, diced

2 or 3 slices goat cheese

3 eggs or 6 quail eggs (higher in nutrition), beaten

Sea salt

Black pepper

Turmeric

Basil leaves

Directions

Preheat a pan with a drizzle of oil. Add the onion and garlic, sauté for a minute, then add the tomatoes, mushrooms, and goat cheese. After a few more minutes, add the eggs and season to taste. Cover the pan with a lid and allow to cook for 5 to 7 minutes. Once ready, dress it up with basil leaves and serve.

Oat Porridge

Ingredients

1 cup rolled oats

1 tablespoon full-fat Greek-style yoghurt

1 teaspoon ground cinnamon

1 teaspoon organic raw peanut butter

Handful fresh or frozen berries

½ banana, sliced

4 or 5 almonds

Directions

Depending on time and wish, you can either cook the oats in a pot for 10 minutes with 1½ cups of water, or cover the oats in boiling water and allow them to soak in the fridge overnight. When your oats are ready, add all the other ingredients, mix well, and enjoy!

Egg Wrap

Ingredients

1 teaspoon olive oil

2 eggs

Wholewheat or rye wrap

½ avocado

1 tablespoon feta cheese

½ large cucumber, cut into cubes

Basil leaves

Turmeric

Coriander

Directions

In a pan, heat the oil and either scramble or fry the eggs. While the eggs are cooking, layer the wrap with the avocado, feta cheese, cucumber, and basil. Add the eggs, and season with turmeric and coriander. Close the wrap and grill, if desired, for 1 to 2 minutes.

Breakfast Bowl

A bowl of whatever was left from last night's dinner (sweet potatoes, green salad) and an addition of fresh morning ingredients.

Ingredients
Sliced avocado
Sliced cucumber
Cut fruit (apple, kiwi, berries, banana)
Handful nuts
2 tablespoons full-fat Greek-style yoghurt
Wholegrain toast with peanut butter

Directions
Put some or all of the ingredients on your plate and enjoy the feast. You deserve it.

Pancakes

Ingredients
2 bananas
500 ml coconut milk
1 cup spelt flour
½ cup rye flour
2 tablespoons honey
2 eggs
Coconut oil, for frying
Maple syrup, fresh fruit, avocado, lemon, for serving

Directions
Combine the bananas, coconut milk, spelt flour, rye flour, honey, and eggs in a blender. Blend to mix well. Heat some oil in a pan

and use the batter to make and cook small pancakes. Serve with maple syrup, fresh fruits, avocado, and lemon.

Acai Bowl

Ingredients
1 banana
½ mango
2 pineapple slices
200 grams frozen acai puree (run in warm water to thaw)
2 tablespoons lemon juice
Toppings: nuts, seeds, ground cinnamon, mint leaves

Directions
Combine the banana, mango, and pineapple in a blender. Blend, then add the acai pure. Blend again, then add the lemon juice. Pour the mixture into a bowl. Top with your desired toppings.

Homemade Granola

This recipe was given to me by my lovely Lina Zoghaib, who is the brightest soul I've ever met. I tried this granola once at her house and immediately announced that it had to be in my next book!

Ingredients
3 cups sesame seeds
1/2 cup flax seeds
1/3 cup chia seeds
1 cup chopped almonds
1 cup organic honey/maple syrup
Zest of 1 orange

Directions

Combine the seeds and almonds in a pan and pan-roast on medium heat for 5 to 8 minutes, stirring. Bring the honey/syrup to a boil in a small saucepan then add the orange zest. Mix immediately with the roasted seeds. Line a flat tray with parchment paper. Pour the mixture onto the tray and tap to level the mixture. Let it rest for 30 minutes then put it in the fridge for 1 hour. Break off pieces with your hand when you want to eat.

Lunch

The secret to always having a healthy filling lunch is to cook a grain of your choice in the morning: quinoa, millet, brown rice, or buckwheat. Apart from rice, they really do take only 15 minutes to cook, whereas rice is best cooked the day before, or you can use leftovers from dinner. Once you have a cooked grain, your imagination can take over and create any salad you want. Open up the fridge, take out some vegetables and herbs, healthy cheeses, even fruit, get your extra-virgin cold-pressed olive oil and some spices, and you're ready to create! Here are some combinations I have created in the past.

Quinoa	Buckwheat	Millet	Brown rice
Iceberg lettuce	Rocket leaves	Parsley	Rocket leaves
Red cabbage	Cucumber	Mango	Avocado
Green apple	Green cabbage	Red onion	Cherry tomatoes
Cherry tomatoes	Avocado	Cucumber	Goat cheese
Cucumber	Blueberries	Iceberg lettuce	Pomegranate seeds
Feta cheese	Cashews	Feta cheese	Walnuts

Try these selections. The quantities are up to you. I want you to sense it yourself and use your intuition. Salad building is a lot of fun and so simple! If you desire an animal protein added to the salad, feel free to do that as well. Once you have your mix together, drizzle it with some olive oil and some lemon juice, add some spices, and that's it! Your lunches have never been so simple, delicious, and nutritious. I look forward to seeing some of your creations on social media!

Dinner

M ost of these recipes are vegetarian; however, if you would like to add some meat or chicken, you can just grill, steam, or roast your preferred animal protein and add it to any of these recipes.

Eggplant and Chickpea Hot Pot
Ingredients
200 grams millet
100 grams raisins, divided
1 tablespoon coconut oil
2 onions, diced
2 to 3 cm fresh ginger, grated
3 garlic cloves, minced
1 medium eggplant, cut into medium chunks
2 teaspoons ground cinnamon
1 teaspoon ground cumin
½ teaspoon paprika
3 tablespoons tomato paste
1 tin organic crushed tomatoes
750 ml vegetable stock, divided
¼ teaspoon saffron
400 grams cooked chickpeas (canned is okay)
Zest and juice of 1 lemon
Pinch sea salt

Directions

Combine the millet and 2 cups of water in a pot. Bring it to a simmer and cook until ready. Add 50 grams of raisins to the millet; use a fork to integrate the raisins and fluff the millet.

Heat the oil in a pan. Add the onions and cook for 1 minute, then add the ginger and garlic. Sauté for 10 minutes until soft. Add the eggplant, cinnamon, cumin, paprika, and tomato paste. Fry for 5 to 6 minutes, adding water if necessary to cool down the heat.

Add the crushed tomatoes, 500 ml of vegetable stock, and the saffron. Stir until it boils and then decrease the heat. Cover with a lid and let it simmer for 30 minutes. Don't forget to stir it occasionally! After 30 minutes, add the chickpeas, the remaining 50 grams of raisins and remaining 250 ml of stock. Let it simmer for another 15 minutes or until the eggplant chunks are soft. Stir in the lemon zest and salt at the end.

To serve, put some millet in a bowl, add a few scoops of your freshly cooked chickpea and eggplant mix, drizzle with some lemon juice, and enjoy with a green salad if desired.

Seabass Pineapple Coconut Curry

Ingredients
1 cup brown rice, rinsed
1 tablespoon coconut oil
2 cm ginger, sliced
1 tablespoon turmeric
5 or 6 pineapple slices, cut into medium chunks

1 cup coconut milk
1 squash, pre-steamed
Steamed seabass

Directions
Combine the rice and 2 cups of water in a pot. Bring it to a simmer and cook until the rice is fully cooked.

While the rice is cooking, heat the oil in a pan, then add the ginger followed by the turmeric. Stir, then add the pineapple. Allow the pineapple chunks to cook a little. Add the coconut milk and squash. Stir the mix gently while it's cooking on low heat.

Add the seabass, season to taste, cook for 5 minutes, and it's ready. Serve on a plate of brown rice. Very rich in flavour! And if you don't want to have fish, then use tofu instead.

Baked Sweet Potato with Vegetable Stuffing

Ingredients
1 large sweet potato, unpeeled (if for one more person, then you need more sweet potatoes!)
Olive oil, for drizzling
1 tablespoon coconut oil or ghee butter
1 onion, diced
1 eggplant, cut into small chunks
½ cup button mushrooms, cut into small chunks
1 red bell pepper, cut into small chunks
Sea salt
Black pepper

Full-fat Greek-style yoghurt
Handful basil leaves

Directions
Preheat the oven to 180°C.

Cut the sweet potato lengthwise, drizzle with olive oil, and bake until very soft.

In a frying pan, heat the coconut oil. Add the onion and sauté for a minute. Then add the eggplant, mushrooms, and bell pepper. Cook until all is soft. Season with sea salt, black pepper, and any other spice you like.

Go back to your sweet potato. Once that's baked and ready, remove the flesh and add it to the veggie mix. Mix well then stuff the sweet potato halves with the mixture, and serve topped with yoghurt and basil leaves.

Baked Vegetables with Brown Rice

A simple yet nutritious recipe! Cook the brown rice while the veggies are baking. It would be great to add avocado-cashew spread here, or just a side of cut cucumbers, cherry tomatoes, and avocado slices drizzled with olive oil.

Ingredients
2 sweet potatoes
3 carrots
2 red bell peppers
1 long zucchini

3 or 4 asparagus spears
Olive oil
Juice of ½ lemon juice
Seasonings: turmeric, sea salt, black pepper, coriander, oregano
3 or 4 garlic cloves
Rosemary sprigs

Directions
Preheat the oven to 180°C. Cut up the sweet potatoes, carrots, bell peppers, zucchini, and asparagus and place on a baking tray. Drizzle with olive oil and the lemon juice, and season with turmeric, salt, pepper, coriander, and oregano. Stir the vegetables on the tray to make sure everything is evenly coated. Place the garlic cloves and rosemary sprigs in the corners of the tray, place the tray in the oven, and bake for 30 minutes or until the sweet potato is soft. Serve with brown rice and a green salad on the side.

Lentil and Sweet Potato Hot Pot

Ingredients
1 tablespoon coconut oil
1 teaspoon ground cumin
1 teaspoon turmeric
1 teaspoon ground coriander
½ teaspoon cayenne pepper
2 cm fresh ginger, grated
4 garlic cloves, minced
1 large red onion, diced
2 sweet potatoes, cut into medium chunks

1 fennel bulb, halved and sliced

200 grams lentils, rinsed

1 litre water

4 tablespoons sauerkraut

2 tablespoons raw honey

Directions

In a large pot, melt the coconut oil. Add the cumin, turmeric, coriander, and cayenne pepper. Stir until fragrant, then add the ginger, garlic, and onion. Carry on cooking for 5 minutes, adding a tablespoon of water if the mixture is getting too dry.

Stir in the sweet potatoes and fennel. Add the lentils and water. Cover with a lid and let it simmer for 25 minutes. Check occasionally, and when the lentils are soft, remove from the heat. Add the sauerkraut and honey, season to taste, and serve in a bowl.

Beetroot Burgers with Lettuce Wraps

Ingredients

4 or 5 raw beets, grated

1 small onion, grated

2 garlic cloves, grated

2 tablespoons olive oil

2 eggs, beaten

150 grams rolled oats

200 grams sheep's cheese or organic firm tofu

1 handful fresh basil leaves

Pinch sea salt

Black pepper

Toppings: lettuce, tomato, avocado, mango, onions

Directions

Combine the beets, onion, and garlic in a large bowl. (You can use a food processor to grate them together or just grate each one by hand.) Add the olive oil, eggs, and oats. Mix everything well then add the cheese or tofu, basil, salt, and pepper, and stir everything well. Set the mixture aside for 30 minutes for the oats to soak and so the patties will hold together.

After 30 minutes, try to form a burger patty. If it's still loose, add more oats. Form the mixture into patties of your preferred size and grill them, or if you're frying, use coconut oil or ghee butter in a frying pan. Cook for a couple of minutes on each side until golden. You can serve the burgers with either lettuce wraps or wholewheat burger buns. I prefer to eat them with lettuce wraps; that way, I can have more than one! Add your desired toppings and enjoy.

Roasted Cauliflower with Buckwheat and Avocado Slices

If you prefer a different whole grain to buckwheat, please go ahead. While you're preparing the cauliflower, you can cook the grain and cut up the avocado slices for the platter.

Ingredients

1 large cauliflower, cut into small/medium florets

1 lime, halved

2 or 3 tablespoons stock or water

1 teaspoon garlic powder

½ teaspoon chili powder

1 teaspoon dried oregano

½ teaspoon ground black pepper

1 or 2 avocados
Olive oil, for drizzling

Directions
Preheat the oven to 230°C. Line a baking tray with parchment paper.

Place the cauliflower florets in a bowl. Squeeze one lime half and reserve the other half. Add the stock or water to the bowl and toss the florets in the liquid. Add the garlic powder, chili powder, oregano, and pepper. Toss well to evenly coat the florets.

Spread the florets and reserved lime half on the baking tray. Place the tray in the oven and roast for 15 to 20 minutes. Toss the florets halfway through the roasting. Once done, they should be slightly crunchy.

Serve with your chosen grain and avocado slices, all drizzled with a bit of olive oil. Perfect meal for dinner!

Snacks

My favourite snack is the almond-cocoa spread, not because I'm a lover of chocolate, but because my partner is, and I found something to suit his sweet tooth! Perhaps it's an idea for you to put a small tub of it into your child's lunchbox with a whole bunch of berries. Delicious!

Roasted Chickpeas

Ingredients
1 cup canned or cooked chickpeas
1 tablespoon olive oil
Seasonings: cayenne pepper, sea salt, turmeric, coriander

Directions
Preheat the oven to 230°C.

In a bowl, mix the chickpeas with the olive oil and seasonings of your preference. Mix well, spread them across a baking tray, and bake in the oven for 30 to 40 minutes. Once ready, store them in an airtight jar and enjoy as a crunchy afternoon snack.

Kale Chips

Ingredients
1 bunch kale, tough stems discarded
1 tablespoon olive oil
1 tablespoon lemon juice
Pinch sea salt

Directions
Preheat the oven to 120°C. Tear the kale leaves into small
pieces, and drizzle with the olive oil, lemon juice, and sea salt.
Massage the kale, making sure every piece is covered in oil,
lemon, and salt. Place on a baking tray and bake in the oven
until crispy, 20 to 30 minutes. Flip them over halfway through
the baking.

Homemade Almond-Cocoa Spread

Ingredients
2 cups dry roasted almonds
1 dark chocolate bar, minimum 75% cocoa
2 teaspoons coconut oil
Pinch sea salt

Directions
In a pot, melt the chocolate together with the coconut oil. In a
food processor, start pulsing the almonds, turning it to a higher
speed to get a butter consistency. Add the chocolate mix and
continue combining while adding sea salt to taste.

Enjoy the chocolate spread on wholegrain toast, in porridge, or
just with berries as a sweet afternoon snack.

Avocado-Cashew Spread

Ingredients

1 cup cashews (soaked overnight, then drained and dried for
15 minutes)

1 avocado

5 or 6 basil leaves

½ teaspoon dried oregano

2 garlic cloves, crushed

Juice of ½ lemon

Juice of ½ lime

Pinch sea salt

Directions

Combine all the ingredients in a food processor or blender and
combine until smooth. Enjoy with veggie sticks for a perfect
nutritious snack!

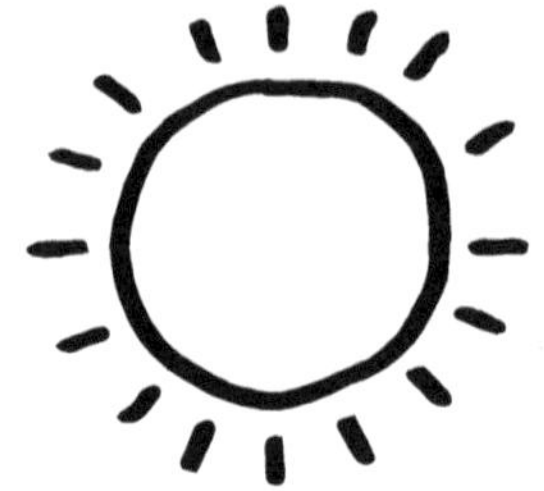

Just when you thought you can never have anything sweet again, Mother Nature has already taken care of it and provided natural "sweet" products.

Baked Goodies

My favourite selection of brownies, muffins, and cookies! It's always nice to make these recipes with others, or even bake them yourself and bring along with you to a social gathering. They will be a hit and you'll be the star of the party. These recipes are very kid-friendly; invite them to mix, fill muffin cups, and anything else you feel your child is able to do. If you have teenagers, they can even be responsible for the whole process, under your supervision.

Avocado Brownies

Ingredients

Coconut oil, for greasing the pan

1 large ripe avocado

2 eggs

½ cup raw honey

1 teaspoon vanilla extract

⅔ cup wholewheat flour (or oat flour/spelt flour)

¼ cup raw cocoa powder

1 teaspoon baking powder

Directions

Preheat the oven to 175°C. Grease a baking pan with coconut oil. The best size of pan would be 9x2 inches, round.

In a blender, combine the avocado, eggs, honey, and vanilla extract. In a separate bowl, whisk together the flour, cocoa powder, and baking powder. Combine the two mixtures and mix well until a batter forms. Pour into the baking pan and bake for about 20 minutes.

Black Bean Cocoa Brownies

Ingredients

125 grams coconut oil

180 grams dark chocolate, minimum 70% cocoa

175 grams cooked black beans

175 grams cooked chickpeas (or canned)

3 tablespoons raw cacao powder

3 tablespoons desiccated coconut powder

120 grams walnuts, roughly chopped

3 eggs

200 ml maple syrup

Pinch sea salt

Directions

Preheat the oven to 175°C. Line a baking tray with parchment paper.

Melt the coconut oil and chocolate in a pan, stirring until fully melted. In a blender or food processor, combine the black beans, chickpeas, cacao powder, coconut powder, and walnuts. Halfway through blending, add the chocolate mixture and continue blending for another minute or so.

In a separate bowl, whisk the eggs for 3 minutes and add the maple syrup and salt. Continue to whisk. Transfer 4 tablespoons of egg mixture to a separate bowl, then add the remaining egg mixture to the chocolate mixture. Mix all nicely and pour into the baking pan. Drip the reserved egg mixture on top of it.

Bake for about 30 minutes, and absolutely wait until the brownie cake has cooled down before cutting.

Banana Muffins with Walnuts

Ingredients
Coconut oil, for greasing muffin cups
1 cup almond flour
1 cup oat flour
2 eggs
½ cup maple syrup
¼ cup water
2 ripe bananas, mashed, plus a few slices
½ cup walnuts, crushed, plus extra
1 teaspoon ground cinnamon
2 teaspoons baking soda
Pinch salt

Directions
Preheat the oven to 170°C. Grease the muffin cups of a muffin tin with coconut oil.

Combine all the ingredients in a bowl. Fill the muffin cups, not too full, and add a few banana slices and crushed walnuts to each muffin cup. Bake for 15 to 20 minutes.

Apple Biscuits

Ingredients

200 grams oat flour

150 grams buckwheat flour

1 teaspoon baking powder

½ teaspoon baking soda

Pinch sea salt

6 tablespoons coconut oil

4 tablespoons almond butter (or peanut butter)

250 ml full-fat Greek-style yoghurt

2 apples, shredded

Directions

Preheat the oven to 230°C. Line a baking tray with parchment paper.

In a large bowl, mix together the flours, baking powder, baking soda, and salt. Add the coconut oil and almond butter and combine everything together with your hands into a pebbly texture. Add the yoghurt and apples and stir with a wooden spoon until you can work the dough by hand. Once the dough forms into a perfect ball, spread it out and cut with a cookie cutter.

Place the biscuits on the baking tray and bake for 15 minutes. Best to eat when still hot!

Homemade pasta

The recipe requires a pasta machine in order to thin the dough. If you do have one, then the rest is easy. This recipe is great for getting the kids to help; it's very safe and fun to play with the dough!

Ingredients
1 cup wholewheat flour
2 eggs
½ teaspoon sea salt

Directions
You can either use your hands or a food processor to make the dough. If by hand, pile the flour on the counter, make a well in the middle, and into the well add the eggs and salt. Slowly start incorporating the eggs with the flour; work with it until it becomes a ball.

If you're using a food processor, combine the flour and salt in the food processor and start pulsing. In a separate bowl, beat the eggs and add them bit by bit to the flour mixture. Process until it turns to a "couscous" texture, then remove and form a ball.

Knead the ball for a good 10 minutes. Once you're done kneading, reshape the dough into a ball, wrap in plastic wrap, cover with a towel, and leave it on the counter for 30 minutes.

Flatten out the dough ball and start taking it through the pasta machine. The process is quite lengthy and requires patience. You have to keep rolling the dough time after time, gradually thinning it until it reaches the thinness you want. Sprinkle it with flour when it gets too sticky.

It's best to eat freshly made pasta on the same day. The first time you try this, it might take some time and confusion; however, you'll soon get better and more familiar with the process. Later on, you can experiment with different flours and make pasta with buckwheat flour, quinoa flour, or any other wholegrain flour. You can also add turmeric or any other favourite spice in the first stages of making the dough, which not only will turn your pasta into a superfood but will also be an awesome colour!

Homemade Milk

The best milk is homemade. When you buy packaged almond milk, you might notice that it's quite diluted, and if you look at the ingredients it has only about 2 percent almonds; the rest is water. Get into the habit of making your own. This recipe is also very kid friendly. Once you teach them the details, they can do it all on their own.

Ingredients
1 cup nuts (almonds, hazelnuts, cashews)
2 cups filtered water
1 teaspoon ground cinnamon

Directions
Soak the nuts overnight. Rinse them the next day, and place in the blender with more filtered water. Blend for a couple of minutes, adding more water if necessary. Place a nut milk bag or cheesecloth over a large jar and pour the blended nut mixture into it. Strain the milk through the nut bag until the pulp is left. Use your hands to squeeze out the last drop of milk. Add the

cinnamon, mix, and pour into an airtight jar. Keep in the fridge and use within 4 to 5 days.

Note: if you get a nut milk machine, you'll just need to add nuts and water and any spices. The machine will do all the work for you.

Sprouts

I enjoy sprouting; it's simple and so rewarding when you eat the delicious results. I also believe that this method is very kid friendly; you can even assign them their own sprouting jar and they become responsible for growing their own vitamins. Let them watch you sprout the first couple of times, and then they'll understand what to expect from this activity: little tails from the little balls!

Any grain, seed, nut, or bean can be sprouted, as long as it hasn't been cooked or roasted. Pick exactly what you would like to sprout, wash 1 cup of it well, and place in a jar. Cover with water to 2 to 3 inches above the grains or seeds. Then cover the jar with a cheesecloth bound by a rubber band, to prevent any insects getting in.

Allow the grains to soak for about 24 hours, then drain the jar and rinse the grains well. Return the grains to the jar, without any water this time. Cover with a cheesecloth bound with a rubber band. Place the jar in a dark corner, and every morning and evening for the next few days, rinse and drain the grains. You'll see little tails growing out of the seeds!

Once they're fully sprouted, you can add them to salads or make a sandwich with avocado and other veggies. Store the sprouted grains in an airtight jar in the fridge.

APPENDIX

The Fructose Content in Fresh Fruits and Dried Fruits from the book *The Sugar Fix* by Dr Richard Johnson.

*Good sources of vitamin C are noted with an asterisk. Vitamin C helps counter the effects of fructose.

Fruit	Serving Size	Grams of Fructose
Fructose Free / Very Low Fructose		
Limes	1 medium	0
Lemons*	1 medium	0.6
Cranberries	1 cup	0.7
Passion Fruit	1 medium	0.9
Low Fructose		
Prune	1 medium	1.2
Apricot	1 medium	1.3

Fruit	Serving Size	Grams of Fructose
Guava	2 medium	2.2
Date (Deglet Noor style)	1 medium	2.6
Plum*	1 medium	2.6
Cantaloupe	⅛ of medium melon	2.8
Raspberries*	1 cup	3.0
Moderate Fructose		
Clementine	1 medium	3.4
Kiwifruit*	1 medium	3.4
Blackberries*	1 cup	3.5
Star fruit	1 medium	3.6
Cherries, sweet	10	3.8
Strawberries*	1 cup	3.8
Cherries, sour	1 cup	4.0
Pineapple*	1 slice	4.0
Grapefruit, pink or red*	½ medium	4.3
Boysenberries	1 cup	4.6

Fruit	Serving Size	Grams of Fructose
Tangerine/mandarin orange*	1 medium	4.8
Nectarine	1 medium	5.4
Peach	1 medium	5.9
Orange (navel)*	1 medium	6.1
Papaya*	½ medium	6.3
Honeydew*	⅛ of medium melon	6.7
Banana	1 medium	7.1
Blueberries	1 cup	7.4
Date (Mejdool)	1 medium	7.7
High Fructose		
Apple	1 medium	9.5
Persimmon	1 medium	10.6
Watermelon	1/16 of medium melon	11.3
Pear	1 medium	11.8
Raisins	¼ cup	12.3
Grapes, seedless (red or green)	1 cup	12.4

Fruit	Serving Size	Grams of Fructose
Mango*	½ medium	16.2
Apricots, dried	1 cup	16.4
Figs, dried	1 cup	23.0

FOOTNOTES & REFERENCES

The Palace Within You

Circle of Life by Institute of Integrative Nutrition

THE KITCHEN

[1] "Heated vegetable oils and cardiovascular disease risk factors" Ng C. Y. et al., NCBI, 2014

[2] "Stop using Canola Oil: 6 Canola oil dangers" Dr Axe, www.draxe.com, 2012

[3] "Olive Oil intake and risk of cardiovascular disease and mortality in the PREDIMED study" Marta Guasch-Ferre et al., NCBI, 2014

[4] "Coconut oil extra-virgin rich diet increases HDL cholesterol and decreases waist circumference in coronary artery disease patients" Cardoso DA et al., NCBI, 2015

[5] Effect of dietary intake of avocado oil and olive oil on biochemical markers of liver function in sucrose-fed rats", Carvajal-Zarrabal O et al., NCBI, 2014

[6] Carotenoid absorption from salad and salsa by humans is enhanced by the addition of avocado or avocado oil", Nuray Z. Unlu et al, Journal of Nutrition, 2005

[7] "How to determine the healthiest fats to cook with?" Dr. Mark Hyman, www.drhyman.com, 2016

[8] "Who is right in the salt debate," Dr Michael Greger, www.nutritionfacts.org, 2018

[9] "Natural sea salt consumption confers protection against hypertension and kidney damage in Dahl salt-sensitive rats," Bog-Hieu Lee et al., NCBI, 2017

[10] "Brain PET imaging in obesity and food addiction," Iozzo P. et al., NCBI, 2012

[11] "Nutrition, non-alcoholic fatty liver and the microbiome: Recent progress in the field," Miriam B. Vis, NCBI, 2015

[12] "The relationship of sugar to population-level diabetes prevalence," Sanjay Basu et al., Journals Plos, 2013

[13] "Soda and cell aging: associations between sugar-sweetened beverage consumption and leukocyte telomere length in healthy adults from the National Health and Nutrition Examination Surveys," C. W. Leung et al., American Journal of Public Health, 2014

[14] "Type 2 diabetes in children: Primary care and public health considerations," Ludwig D. S., Ebbeling C. B., NCBI, 2001

[15] David Tong MD, American Stroke Association, Annual Meeting, 2011 (abstract)

[16] "According to National Nutrient Database for Standard Reference 1 Release April 2018," www.ndb.nal.usda.gov

[17] "The Sugar Fix," Dr Richard Johnson

[18] "Effect of honey consumption on plasma antioxidant status in human subjects," Gross H, News Release, 2002

[19] "Health Benefits of Manuka Honey as an essential constituent for tissue regeneration," Niaz K. et al., NCIB, 2017

[20] "Oats and Buckwheat intakes and cardiovascular disease risk factors in an ethnic minority in China," He J. et al., NCBI, 1995

[21] "Effects of high-bran bread on glucose control in insulin dependent diabetic patients," Nygren C. et al., Europe PMC, 1984

[22] "Coconut fats," Amarasiri W. A. et al., NCBI, 2006

23 "Nutritional improvements of cereals by sprouting," Chavan J. K., NCBI, 1989

24 "Replacing white rice with brown rice or other whole grains may reduce the risk of diabetes," Press Release, Harvard School of Public Health, 2010

25 "Arsenic in your food," Consumer Reports, www.consumerreports.org, 2012

26 "Milk stimulates the growth of prostate cancer cells in culture," Tate P. L. et al., NCBI, 2011

27 "Coconut milk nutrition," Dr Axe, www.draxe.com, 2015

28 "Almond milk: a potential therapeutic weapon against cow's milk protein allergy," Cuppari C. et al., NCBI, 2015

29 "Effectiveness of probiotics in irritable bowel syndrome: updated systematic review with meta-analysis," World Journal of Gastroenterology, 2015

30 "Is cheese bad for you? Top 5 healthiest cheese options and benefits," Dr. Axe, www.draxe.com, 2018

31 According to the National Cancer Institute, 2017

32 "Epidemiology of Type 1 Diabetes," David M. Maahs et al., NCBI, 2011

33 "Methemoglobinemia from eating meat with high nigh nitrite content," J. D. Orgeron, NCBI, 1957

34 "IARC Monographs evaluate consumption of red meat and processed meat," International Agency for Research on Cancer, WHO, 2015

35 "Nitrosamine exposure causes Insulin Resistance Diseases," Ming Tong et al., NCBI, 2010

36 "A history of pesticide use," Patricia S. Muir, Oregon State University, 2012

37 "2018 Dirty Dozen Report," Environmental Working Group, 2018

THE BATHROOM

[1] "Triclosan-containing antibacterial soaps neither safe nor effective," Report by Environmental Working Group, 2014

[2] "Should people be concerned about Parabens in their beauty product?" Press Release, Scientific American, 2010

[3] "Is your toothpaste loaded with toxins?" Dr. Mercola, www.articles.mercola.com, 2016

[4] "Tumorigenic effect of commonly used moisturising creams when applies topically to UVB pre-treated high-risk mice," Yao-Ping Lu et al, NCBI, 2009

[5] "5 things wrong with your deodorant," Heid M., Time Magazine, 2016

[6] "The health risks of secret chemicals in fragrance."

[7] The Campaign for Safe Cosmetics by Environmental Working Group, 2010

"Non-toxic nail polishes anything but non-toxic," Report by Environmental Working Group, 2012

[8] "Can hair-dye give you cancer?", Dr. Mercola, www.articles.mercola.com, 2008

"Lead and other heavy metals"

[9] Campaign for Safe Cosmetics, www.safecosmetics.org, 2018

[10] "EWG's Sunscreen Guide," Environmental Working Group, 2018

CLEAN YOUR HOME WITH CLEAN PRODUCTS

[1] "WHO releases country estimates on air pollution exposure and health impact," News Release, WHO, 2016

[2] "Cleaning at home and at work in relation to lung function decline and airway obstruction," American Journal of Respiratory and Critical Care Medicine, 2017

[3] "The long-term effects of cleaning on the lungs," Kristin J. Cummings et al, American Journal of Respiratory and Critical Care Medicine, 2018

[4] "Your laundry detergent may contain toxic ingredients," Dr Mercola, www.articles.mercola.com, 2011

WAYS TO ENHANCE YOUR HOME

[1] "Health effects of Microwave radiation – Microwave Ovens," Lita Lee Ph.D, PubMed, 1998

[2] "Effects of Microwave Radiation on anti-infective factors in human milk", R Quan, PubMed, 1992

[3] "Essential Oils" by Makus Shirner, Shirner Publishing House, 2005

[4] "Candles and Incense as potential sources of indoor air pollution," Environmental Protection Agency, USA, 2001

[5] Microwave Frequency Electromagnetic Fields produce widespread neuropsychiatric effects including depression," Journal of Chemical Neuroanatomy, Martin Pall 2016

[6] Ibid (same as above)

[7] "Plastic Pollution: how humans are turning the world into plastic," UN Environment Program, 2018

[8] "A sperm whale that washed up on a beach in Spain had 64 pounds of plastic and waste in its stomach," Andrea Diaz, CNN, 2018

RECIPE SECTION

page 179: Adopted from Green Kitchen App (available on IOS only)

page 183: Adopted and slightly altered from Green Kitchen App

page 184: Adopted and slightly altered from Green Kitchen App

page 185: Adopted from Rouxbe Culinary School

page 188: Adopted from Rouxbe Culinary School

page 189: Adopted from Rouxbe Culinary School

page 191: Adopted and slightly altered from David Avocado Wolfe Recipes

page 192: Adopted from Green Kitchen App

page 193: Adopted from Green Kitchen App

page 194: Adopted and slightly altered from Dr Axe Recipes

page 195: Adopted from Green Kitchen App

Rouxbe Culinary School

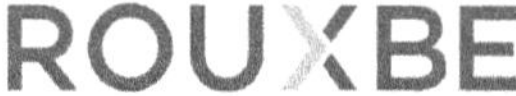

You can cut this page out of the book and use the Circle of Life to measure your progress. Mark a dot on each line of each life element to indicate your level of satisfaction. Placing a dot closer to the centre of the circle shows dissatisfaction, whereas placing a dot toward the periphery shows satisfaction. As a last step, connect the dots to see how balanced you are in your life.

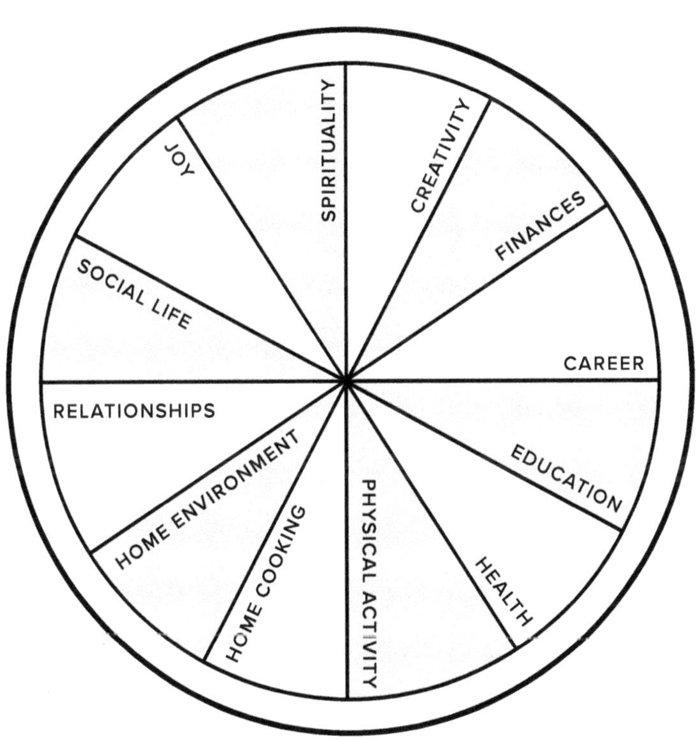

ACKNOWLEDGEMENTS

When I was young, I always imagined myself doing something grand. I had, and still have, a book of dreams in which I would draw or write my dream projects, my dream life. And every month, I had something different. I went from owning a huge multinational logistic company that would transport goods underground at bullet speed, to starting a beauty salon with patented chocolate face masks, to being a dancer, then a model, to starting a cultural school in China to help kids settle in when they study abroad, to having my own retreat centre sustained by an organic farm next door and also opening several orphanages across the world. But never did I imagine that by the age of thirty, I would have written two books, travelled on book tours, held international yoga retreats, consulted over a hundred people on their health, and transformed their lives toward better. Even though my teenage dreams weren't aligned with the present moment, there's one thing in common: I knew I had a purpose. I knew I was up for an adventure.

Everybody has a purpose. Sometimes, it's difficult to realise that, and when you do, it's challenging to identify what it is and then, it isn't easy at all to follow your "purpose" due to the bills you have to pay!

When I sat to write this Acknowledgement section, I really just wanted to appreciate the hard work I've been putting into my growth. This may sound self-centred and egoistic, but that isn't the intention. So many of us forget to praise, appreciate, and acknowledge our own self. We're working so hard and then wait for the appreciation and respect of our family, friends, clients, managers, readers, competitors, societies, and the rest of the world. We tend to feel very good when we receive that praise from outside. It's uncommon or, in some cases, even frowned upon to take a moment and say "I'm so proud of myself. If it weren't for my hard work, for my creative thinking, for my kindness, for my ..., I wouldn't be where I am today." Of course, Life gives you support and opportunities, but it's how you treat these gifts from Life.

I'm very thankful for everything that has been given to me in order for me to be where I am, yet I'm even more thankful for my discipline, hard work, and determination to live my purpose. In movies, you see authors isolating themselves to write in nice country houses with a beautiful view on to lakes and forests. I wish that had been my reality; instead, I was juggling family commitments, client commitments, nourishing myself, exercising, being there for my partner and my dogs, yet the book had to be finished. I was up typing away at 5 a.m. for a couple of hours before the world woke up and sucked me into the routine. I was typing during lunch breaks and just before falling asleep. I didn't stop; I couldn't because the reason behind writing was too grand to stop.

I knew it back then when I was fifteen, and I know it very well today, fifteen years later: I have a purpose. Today, I'm just very grateful to myself for following that purpose against all the odds. And I would like to acknowledge that.

This isn't your typical Acknowledgement section, but take a moment here. Close your eyes, take a deep breath in and out, and acknowledge yourself for everything you are.

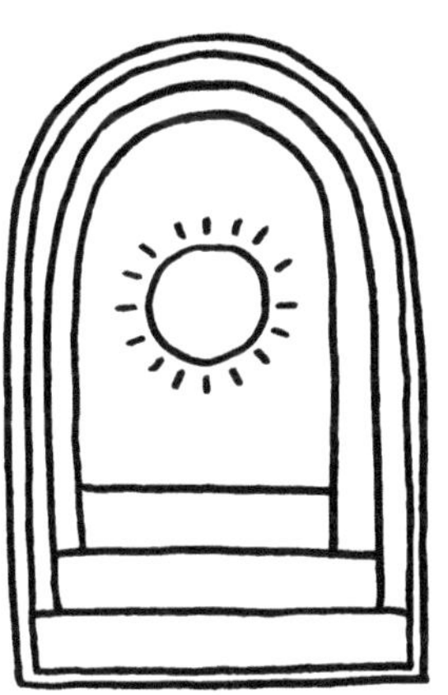

CPSIA information can be obtained
at www.ICGtesting.com
Printed in the USA
LVHW020245170721
692932LV00011B/971